WORKBOOK TO ACCOMPANY

HUMAN DISEASES

Fourth Edition

Marianne Neighbors, EdD, RN
Professor Emeritus
Eleanor Mann School of Nursing
University of Arkansas
Fayetteville, Arkansas

Ruth Tannehill-Jones, MS, RN
Former Chief Clinical Officer Regency Hospital
Vice President Patient Care Services Mercy Hospital
Northwest Arkansas

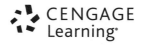
CENGAGE
Learning®

Australia • Brazil • Japan • Korea • Mexico • Singapore • Spain • United Kingdom • United States

CENGAGE
Learning®

Workbook to Accompany Human Diseases, Fourth Edition
Marianne Neighbors and Ruth Tannehill-Jones

Vice President/General Manager, Skills and Product Planning: Dawn Gerrain

Product Director, Health Care Skills: Stephen Helba

Product Team Manager: Matthew Seeley

Senior Director, Development: Marah Bellegarde

Product Development Manager, Health Care Skills: Juliet Steiner

Senior Content Developer, Health Care Skills: Debra M. Myette-Flis

Product Assistant: Melanie Chapman

Marketing Brand Manager: Wendy Mapstone

Senior Production Director: Wendy Troeger

Production Manager: Andrew Crouth

Content Project Manager: Thomas Heffernan

Senior Art Director: Jack Pendleton

Cover image(s): iStock.com/traffic_analyzer

For product information and technology assistance, contact us at
Cengage Learning Customer & Sales Support, 1-800-354-9706
For permission to use material from this text or product, submit all requests online at **www.cengage.com/permissions.**
Further permissions questions can be e-mailed to
permissionrequest@cengage.com

Library of Congress Control Number: 2013948334

ISBN-13: 978-1-285-06593-9

Cengage Learning
200 First Stamford Place, 4th Floor
Stamford, CT 06902
USA

Cengage Learning is a leading provider of customized learning solutions with office locations around the globe, including Singapore, the United Kingdom, Australia, Mexico, Brazil, and Japan. Locate your local office at: **www.cengage.com/global**

Cengage Learning products are represented in Canada by Nelson Education, Ltd.

To learn more about Cengage Learning, visit **www.cengage.com**

Purchase any of our products at your local college store or at our preferred online store **www.cengagebrain.com**

Printed in the United States of America
2 3 4 5 6 7 16 15

CONTENTS

Human Diseases, Fourth Edition, helps you learn basic disease information. Organized by body systems, this essential pathophysiology text is written specifically for allied health learners and as a reference for allied health professionals. This book is also ideal as a resource on basic diseases by anyone within the medical arena or lay community. It is designed to make difficult pathophysiology concepts easier to understand by using consistent organization, and it includes pronunciations, boxed features, and full-color illustrations and photos. Chapters progress through a basic review of anatomy and physiology before introducing the most common diseases. Common diseases and disorders are presented consistently through description, etiology, symptoms, diagnosis, treatment, and prevention headings.

TO THE LEARNER

Each chapter in the workbook corresponds to the same chapter in the book. A variety of exercises are included to help reinforce the material you learned in the book. Types of exercises include matching terms; completion; short answer; true/false; define terms; define abbreviations; identify diagnostic tests; and condition tables.

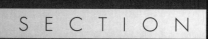
Concepts of Human Diseases

Introduction to Human Diseases

Define Terms

Define the following terms:

1. acute_____

   _____

2. auscultation _____

   _____

3. diagnosis _____

   _____

4. etiology _____

   _____

5. nosocomial _____

   _____

6. palliative _____

   _____

7. palpation _____

   _____

8. pathologic _____

   _____

9. symptom _____

   _____

10. mortality _____

    _____

Matching Terms

Match the following terms with the correct definition:

_____ 1. chronic

_____ 2. complication

_____ 3. exacerbation

_____ 4. homeostasis

_____ 5. pathogens

A. symptoms flare-up or become worse

B. a state of sameness

C. a disease that persists for a long time

D. the onset of a second disease or disorder

E. removing a small piece of tissue for examination

F. microorganisms that cause disease

Match the following terms with the correct definition:

_____ 6. remission

_____ 7. pathologic

_____ 8. disease

_____ 9. preventive

_____ 10. prognosis

A. predicted or expected outcome of the disease

B. the study of tumors

C. a change in structure or function

D. a time when symptoms are diminished

E. something that reduces risk

F. caused by a disease

Define Abbreviations

Define the following abbreviations:

1. CBC _____

2. UA _____

3. EKG or ECG _____

4. CXR _____

5. CAT _____

Identify Diagnostic Tests

Define the following diagnostic tests:

1. complete blood count _____

2. urinalysis _____

3. electrocardiography _____

4. blood glucose _____

5. computerized axial tomography _____

Completion

Using the words in the list, complete the following statements:

acute	homeostasis
chronic	nosocomial
iatrogenic	palliative
diagnosis	predisposing factors
exacerbations	prognosis
holistic medicine	remission

1. _____ care is aimed at preventing pain and discomfort but does not seek to cure the disease.

2. The state of sameness or normalcy is known as _____.

3. A time when symptoms are diminished or temporarily resolved is called _____.

4. A condition that is short term with a sudden onset is called _____.

5. A problem arising from a prescribed treatment is called _____.

6. Risk factors are also called _____.

7. _____ is the predicted or expected outcome.

8. Flare-ups (the return of symptoms) are _____.

9. When the physician identifies or names a disease identified in a patient, it is called the patient's _____.

10. Diabetes is a _____ disease because it lasts for a long or extended period of time.

11. A disease acquired from the hospital environment is called _____.

12. The concept where the whole person, rather than just the physical being, is considered is known as _____ medicine.

Short Answer

Provide answers to the following:

1. Define *predisposing* factors.

_____

_____

_____

_____

2. List some predisposing factors.

a. _____

b. _____

c. _____

d. _____

e. _____

3. Explain the difference between a disorder and a syndrome.

_____

_____

_____

_____

4. Describe the pathogenesis of a disease.

_____

_____

_____

_____

True/False

____ 1. When using good hand-washing techniques, you should use an antimicrobial soap.

____ 2. It is important to use a fingernail cleaner whenever possible if you are following good hand-washing protocol.

____ 3. When washing the hands, after soaping and rubbing them, you should rinse starting from the wrist then over the fingertips.

____ 4. The use of standard precautions is only recommended by the Centers for Disease Control and Prevention when administering care to a patient who is bleeding or has other body fluid discharge.

____ 5. A hypodermic needle should never be recapped.

CASE STUDY

Emily is a 25-year-old Asian female. Emily is complaining of frequent headaches over the past 3 weeks. Emily is taking birth control pills and smokes one package of cigarettes a day. She complains of severe head pain, light sensitivity, nausea, and vomiting. She has had no relief from over-the-counter medications such as Tylenol or ibuprofen.

Using the information from the case study, list a possible diagnosis, risk factors, symptoms, and the etiology.

_____

_____

_____

_____

CHAPTER 2

Mechanisms of Disease

Define Terms

Define the following terms:

1. congenital _____

_____

2. infection _____

_____

3. neoplasm _____

_____

4. malignant _____

_____

5. allergy _____

_____

6. cancer _____

_____

7. disease _____

_____

8. metastatic _____

_____

9. acute _____

_____

10. trauma _____

_____

Matching Terms

Match the following terms with the correct definition:

_____ 1. hypertrophy   A. naming or identifying a disease

_____ 2. atrophy   B. increase in size or growth

_____ 3. diagnosis   C. without growth or decrease in cell size

_____ 4. gangrene   D. hypoxia of cells

_____ 5. ischemia   E. necrotic tissue attacked by saprophytic bacteria

                              F. enclosed in a capsule

Match the following terms with the correct definition:

_____ 6. infarct

_____ 7. hypoxia

_____ 8. cachexia

_____ 9. antibodies

_____ 10. inflammation

A. a protective response triggered by injury

B. necrosis of cells due to ischemia

C. proteins that react to antigens

D. ill, thin, wasted appearance

E. related to the small intestine

F. not enough oxygen in cells

Define Abbreviations

Define the following abbreviations:

1. TPN _____

2. AIDS _____

3. MVA _____

Completion

Using the words in the list, complete the following statements:

anoxia

benign

degenerative diseases

hypoxia

infarct

-itis

malignant

trauma

1. Diseases that are related to inflammation are identified by the suffix _____.

2. Neoplasms can be classified as _____ and _____.

3. Cellular injury and death may be due to _____, _____, or _____, or toxins or viruses.

4. When necrosis occurs due to ischemia, the area of dead cells is an _____.

5. Diseases related to aging may be called _____.

Short Answer

Provide answers to the following:

1. List the classification groups for trauma.

   _____

   _____

   _____

2. State some examples of causes of diseases.

   _____

   _____

   _____

3. Describe the following neoplasms:

adenoma _____

carcinoma _____

fibroma _____

glioma _____

lipoma _____

melanoma _____

sarcoma _____

4. Describe the changes in the body occurring in the aging process.

_____

_____

_____

5. What are the common ways the immune system may malfunction?

_____

_____

_____

6. List two ways the immune system protects the body.

_____

_____

_____

7. What factors affect the aging process?

a. _____

b. _____

c. _____

d. _____

e. _____

8. What conditions are necessary for a cell to survive?

a. _____

b. _____

c. _____

9. List the different types of cell adaptation.

a. _____

b. _____

c. _____

d. _____

e. _____

f. _____

10. What are the three different types of gangrene?

a. _____

b. _____

c. _____

True/False

_____ 1. It is important to eat only small amounts of fiber in the daily diet.

_____ 2. No more than one alcohol drink per day for females and two for males is the recommended daily allowance for a healthy lifestyle.

_____ 3. Only moderate or small amounts of fat intake per day are recommended.

_____ 4. More consumers are seeking health knowledge via the Internet.

_____ 5. Consumers should be more educated about their health status and their medications.

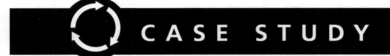

CASE STUDY

Jonathan is a 29-year-old diesel mechanic. Because of the high cost of gasoline, Jonathan has been riding his motorcycle rather than driving his half-ton pickup back and forth to work in order to save money. The temperature is 95°F, so Jonathan decides not to wear his helmet on his way home from work. One mile down the freeway, Jonathan changes lanes and is hit by a car. He sustains a severe head injury. He is transported to the local hospital and admitted to the intensive care unit. Jonathan is unresponsive.

What criteria will be used to determine if Jonathan is brain dead?

_____

_____

_____

_____

Neoplasms

Define Terms

Define the following terms:

1. benign _____

   _____

2. cachexia _____

   _____

3. cytology _____

   _____

4. hematoma _____

   _____

5. malignant _____

   _____

6. metastasis _____

   _____

7. neoplasm _____

   _____

8. palliative _____

   _____

9. preventive _____

   _____

10. tumor _____

    _____

Matching Terms

Match the following terms with the correct definition:

____ 1. biopsy

____ 2. carcinoma

____ 3. curative

____ 4. dysplasia

____ 5. frozen section

A. removing a small piece of tissue for microscopic examination

B. something that corrects the disease or condition

C. determining the degree of differentiation of cells by microscopic examination

D. neoplasm arising from epithelial tissue

E. technique that allows rapid diagnosis

F. an alteration in size, shape, and organization of cells

Match the following terms with the correct definition:

____ 6. grading

____ 7. hyperplasia

____ 8. radiation

____ 9. sarcoma

____ 10. staging

A. an increase in cell number

B. the process of using light, short waves or X-rays

C. neoplasm arising from connective tissue or bone

D. determining the degree of spread of a malignant tumor

E. a new growth

F. determining the degree of differentiation of cells by microscopic examination

Identify Signs and Symptoms of Cancer

Identify how the following may be signs or symptoms of cancer:

1. pain _____

2. obstruction _____

3. hemorrhage _____

4. anemia _____

5. fracture _____

6. infection _____

7. cachexia _____

Identify Diagnostic Tests

Match the following terms with the correct definition:

____ 1. screening

____ 2. occult stool

____ 3. annual physical examination

____ 4. cancer warning signals

____ 5. Pap test

____ 6. biopsy

____ 7. frozen section

A. microscopic examination that allows rapid diagnosis

B. earlier testing for disease; a measure such as monthly breast examinations

C. live tissue examination

D. yearly examination by physician

E. acronym CAUTION

F. staining test often used for cervical cytology

G. test to screen for colon cancer

Completion

Using the words in the list, complete the following statements:

angiogenesis   cytology

biopsy   grading

carcinogens   hematoma

carcinoma in situ   staging

chemotherapy   tumors

1. _____ determines the degree of abnormality of the neoplasm.

2. A large tumor or swelling filled with blood, commonly called a bruise or contusion, is also known as a _____.

3. Neoplasms are commonly called _____.

4. Cancer-causing agents are known as _____.

5. _____ considers the degree of spread.

6. Removing a small piece of tissue for microscopic examination is known as a _____.

7. _____ is the examination of cells.

8. Atypical cells that just sit in the epithelial layer of tissue and have not broken through the basement membrane are called _____.

9. New growth of blood vessels is called _____.

10. _____ is the use of medications to kill or inhibit the growth of neoplasms.

Short Answer

Provide answers to the following:

1. Compare benign tumors to malignant tumors.

   _____

   _____

   _____

2. Explain the system used to classify neoplasms.

   _____

   _____

   _____

3. There are several factors that regulate the growth of normal cells. List them.

   a. _____

   b. _____

   c. _____

4. Describe a metastatic neoplasm.

   _____

   _____

   _____

5. What causes genetic mutation?

    a. _____

    b. _____

    c. _____

    d. _____

6. List the personal risk behaviors that put an individual at increased risk for developing cancer.

    a. _____

    b. _____

    c. _____

    d. _____

7. List the factors that decrease a female's risk for developing breast cancer.

    a. _____

    b. _____

    c. _____

8. Increased consumption of what dietary items is considered preventive in cancer development?

    a. _____

    b. _____

    c. _____

9. What are the American Cancer Society's recommendations for cancer prevention?

    a. _____

    b. _____

    c. _____

    d. _____

    e. _____

    f. _____

    g. _____

    h. _____

    i. _____

10. What does the acronym CAUTION stand for?

    C _____

    A _____

    U _____

    T _____

    I _____

    O _____

    N _____

11. What are the three major types of cancer treatment?

a. _____

b. _____

c. _____

True/False

_____ 1. Beginning in their 20s, women should be made aware of the benefits and limitations of breast self-examinations (BSEs).

_____ 2. Finding a change in breast tissue means that cancer is present.

_____ 3. Researchers are testing the effectiveness of dendritic cell vaccines for preventing tumor growth and extending life in patients with cancer.

_____ 4. Dendritic cells occur naturally in tissues such as the skin and the lining of nose, lungs, stomach, and intestines.

_____ 5. Some studies have shown that alternative therapies used as the main treatment for breast cancer may result in increased recurrence of the disease and even death.

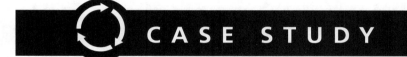

CASE STUDY

Susan is a 52-year-old elementary school teacher. Her sister (age 47) was recently diagnosed with metastatic breast cancer. Susan has yearly clinical breast examinations and a mammogram but has never done a breast self-examination (BSE).

Describe the process of BSE as if you were explaining it to Susan.

_____

_____

_____

_____

CHAPTER 4

Inflammation and Infection

Define Terms

Define the following terms:

1. bacteria _____

_____

2. trauma _____

_____

3. hyperemia _____

_____

4. adhesion _____

_____

5. odoriferous _____

_____

6. septicemia _____

_____

7. pus _____

_____

8. lesion _____

_____

9. scab _____

_____

10. purulent _____

_____

Matching Terms

Match the following terms with the correct definition:

_____ 1. pyogenic

_____ 2. abscess

_____ 3. cellulitis

_____ 4. fistula

_____ 5. keloid

A. a tract that connects two organs

B. movement of cells in response to chemicals

C. pus forming

D. excessive collagen formation

E. a localized collection of pus

F. inflammation of connective tissue

Match the following terms with the correct definition:

_____ 6. ulcer

_____ 7. infection

_____ 8. exudate

_____ 9. malaise

_____ 10. empyema

A. a crater-like lesion in the skin

B. a process of washing away necrotic tissue

C. fluid that seeps out of tissue or capillaries

D. invasion of microorganisms into tissue

E. an accumulation of pus in a body cavity

F. general ill feeling

Completion

Using the words in the list, complete the following statements:

abscesses

adhesions

cellulitis

dehiscence

inflammation

keloid

mast cells

primary union

skin testing

ulcers

1. _____ are also called tissue histiocytes.

2. _____ is the nonspecific cellular and vascular reaction to tissue trauma.

3. Inflammatory lesions include _____, _____, and _____.

4. Healing by first intention is also called _____ _____.

5. Separation of tissue margins is called _____.

6. Excessive collagen formation often results in a hard, raised scar called a _____.

7. Fibrous bands that develop as a complication of surgery are called _____.

8. _____ may be used to determine the presence of exposure to a pathogen like tuberculosis.

Short Answer

Provide answers to the following:

1. Describe the basic defense mechanisms in the body that help prevent infections.

_____

_____

_____

2. Explain the steps in wound healing.

_____

_____

_____

3. List some common infectious microorganisms.

_____

_____

_____

4. What are the three primary goals of the inflammatory response?

    a. _____

    b. _____

    c. _____

5. What are the "foot soldiers" of the inflammatory process?

_____

_____

_____

6. Describe a lesion.

    a. _____

    b. _____

7. List three inflammatory lesions.

    a. _____

    b. _____

    c. _____

8. How is an abscess formed?

_____

_____

_____

9. List three examples of an abscess.

    a. _____

    b. _____

    c. _____

10. What are the signs of acute inflammation?

    a. _____

    b. _____

    c. _____

    d. _____

11. What happens when an ulcer is formed?

    a. _____

    b. _____

12. What are the characteristics of cellulitis?

_____

_____

_____

13. What are the causes of cellulitis?

    a. _____

    b. _____

    c. _____

14. How is cellulitis typically treated?

_____

_____

_____

15. What is the function of a scab?

_____

_____

_____

16. What is an opportunistic infection?

_____

_____

_____

17. Where do bacteria normally live?

    a. _____

    b. _____

    c. _____

    d. _____

    e. _____

18. What does the abbreviation MRSA stand for?

_____

_____

_____

19. List common infections caused by the bacterium *Streptococcus*.

    a. _____

    b. _____

    c. _____

    d. _____

20. What immunizations are effective in preventing viral infections?

    a. _____

    b. _____

    c. _____

    d. _____

    e. _____

21. List four common fungal infections.

    a. _____

    b. _____

    c. _____

    d. _____

True/False

_____ 1. Once an individual no longer has pain or drainage in an infection site, it is okay to stop taking the prescribed antibiotics.

_____ 2. Good hand washing is the best preventive measure against the common cold.

CASE STUDY

Stephen, age 17, developed a rash and possible skin infection on his arms and torso. He has had a cold for a couple of weeks and has also had an elevated temperature at times. He was not concerned about the cold, but since he developed the rash with some draining vesicles, he has become very anxious about the problem. His mother made an appointment for him to see his primary care physician since she is worried that he has developed an infection along with the rash.

1. List some symptoms of infection.

_____

_____

2. What diagnostic tests might Stephen's physician use to determine if he has an infection?

_____

_____

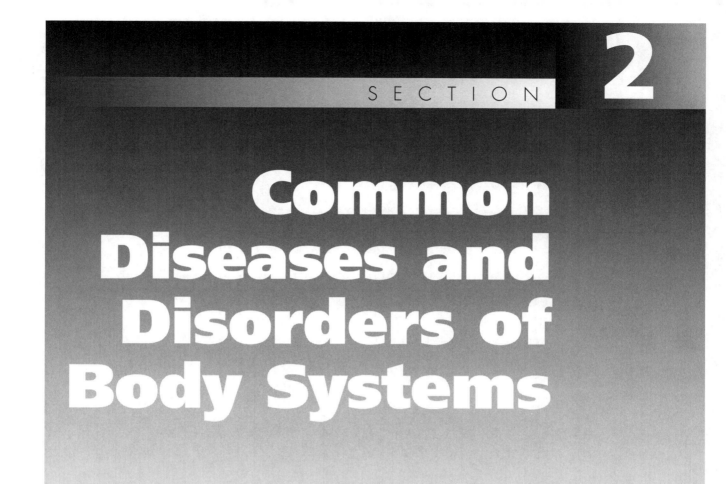

Common Diseases and Disorders of Body Systems

CHAPTER 5

Immune System Diseases and Disorders

Define Terms

Define the following terms:

1. allergy _____

_____

2. streptococcal _____

_____

3. prophylactic _____

_____

4. bronchospasm _____

_____

5. allergen _____

_____

Matching Terms

Match the following terms with the correct definition:

____	1. autoimmune	A. hives
____	2. antigen	B. RF
____	3. hemolytic	C. immunity against self
____	4. rheumatoid factor	D. destroys blood
____	5. urticaria	E. cell marker that causes a state of sensitivity to an antibody
		F. dry eyes

Match the following terms with the correct definition:

____	6. immunodeficiency	A. lack of immunity
____	7. ptosis	B. severe allergic reaction
____	8. cytotoxic	C. cell killing
____	9. anaphylaxis	D. double vision
____	10. diplopia	E. immunity against self
		F. drooping eyelids

Identify Diagnostic Tests

Fill in the blanks with the correct terms:

1. The most important test for diagnosing allergies is _____.

2. The test that indicates the formation of antibodies on the red blood cell is the _____.

3. Autoimmune disorders may be diagnosed utilizing _____ tests that measure for specific diseases.

4. Finding an antibody against the human immunodeficiency virus (HIV) is indicative of exposure to _____.

Condition Table

Complete the following table:

Condition and Definition	Signs and Symptoms	Diagnostic Tests	Treatment Plan
Hay Fever			
Asthma			
Urticaria			
Anaphylaxis			
Contact Dermatitis			
Rheumatic Fever			
Rheumatoid Arthritis			
Myasthenia Gravis			
Lupus Erythematosus			
Scleroderma			
Blood Transfusion Reaction			
Organ Rejection			
AIDS			

Completion

Using the words in the list, complete the following statements:

acetylcholine	itching
anaphylaxis	lymphocytes
antigens	redness
diffuse	self-antigen
discoid	swelling
heat	T cells
human immunodeficiency virus	thymus
hypersensitivity disorder	
inflammation	
isoimmune disorder	

1. _____ are the major cells of the immune system.

2. _____, _____, _____, and _____ are common inflammatory responses to allergic reactions.

3. The result of an overreaction of the immune system to an antigen is called a _____ _____.

4. _____ is a severe allergic response to an allergen.

5. Autoimmune disorders are hypersensitivities in which the body fails to recognize its own _____.

6. Rheumatoid arthritis begins with _____ of the synovial lining of a joint.

7. Myasthenia gravis disrupts the transmission of _____, which affects the nerve impulses going to the muscles.

8. The two types of lupus erythematosus include _____ and _____.

9. _____ refers to a hypersensitivity of one person to another person's tissue.

10. _____ on the red blood cells give each type of cell a special identity.

11. The cause of AIDS is a _____ _____ _____.

12. As the _____ gland decreases in size with aging, so does the number of _____.

Short Answer

Provide answers to the following:

1. What are the primary and secondary organs of the immune system?

   a. _____

   b. _____

   c. _____

   d. _____

   e. _____

   f. _____

2. List the cells of the immune system.

   a. _____

   b. _____

   c. _____

   d. _____

   e. _____

3. Name two types of immune responses.

   a. _____

   b. _____

4. List the different types of immunity and give an example of each type.

   a. _____

   b. _____

   c. _____

   d. _____

5. What is natural immunity?

   _____

   _____

   _____

6. What is the clinical problem associated with immune deficiency disorders?

   _____

   _____

   _____

7. What are the two main groups of diseases of the immune system?

   a. _____

   b. _____

8. List the signs and symptoms of allergies.

   a. _____

   b. _____

   c. _____

   d. _____

   e. _____

   f. _____

   g. _____

9. Define status asthmaticus.

   _____

   _____

10. What are the triggers for nonallergic asthma?

    a. _____

    b. _____

    c. _____

    d. _____

11. What substances commonly cause anaphylactic reactions?

    a. _____

    b. _____

    c. _____

    d. _____

    e. _____

    f. _____

    g. _____

    h. _____

    i. _____

    j. _____

    k. _____

    l. _____

12. What are the symptoms of food allergies?

    a. _____

    b. _____

    c. _____

13. What allergens are common causes of contact dermatitis?

    a. _____

    b. _____

    c. _____

    d. _____

    e. _____

    f. _____

    g. _____

14. What are autoimmune disorders?

    _____

    _____

    _____

15. List some examples of autoimmune disorders.

    a. _____

    b. _____

    c. _____

    d. _____

    e. _____

16. When does acute organ rejection occur?

    _____

    _____

    _____

17. What is an immunodeficiency disorder?

    _____

    _____

    _____

18. How is immune deficiency acquired?

    a. _____

    b. _____

    c. _____

19. What commonly leads to immunodeficiency?

    a. _____

    b. _____

    c. _____

    d. _____

20. List the five stages of HIV.

    a. _____

    b. _____

    c. _____

    d. _____

    e. _____

21. List the three primary ways HIV can be spread or transmitted.

    a. _____

    b. _____

    c. _____

True/False

_____ 1. Research has shown that T cells play an important role in protecting the body from infectious diseases.

_____ 2. The immune system is important in preserving the body's immunity by eliminating tumors that produce antigens.

_____ 3. Research has shown that borage oil might be effective for treating rheumatoid arthritis, but it may also cause serious side effects.

_____ 4. Diseases of the immune system are usually divided into four main groups.

_____ 5. Research has shown that caution should be used when taking alternative medicines for treatment of rheumatoid arthritis.

_____ 6. Most treatment related to AIDS has been life-saving.

_____ 7. One strategy to prevent AIDS transmission is to be sure to use birth control pills when engaging in sexual intercourse.

_____ 8. A recommended strategy to prevent AIDS transmission is to refrain from having multiple sex partners or having sex with intravenous drug users.

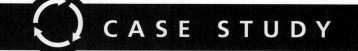

CASE STUDY

Jason, age 10, was brought to the emergency room by his mother. He had been stung by a bee and was having some difficulty in breathing. She thought he might be having an anaphylactic reaction.

1. What are the symptoms of a localized anaphylactic reaction?

_____

_____

2. What are the symptoms of a systemic anaphylactic reaction?

_____

_____

3. What is the treatment for an anaphylactic reaction?

_____

_____

_____

CHAPTER 6

Musculoskeletal System Diseases and Disorders

Define Terms

Define the following terms:

1. fascia _____

   _____

2. interphalangeal _____

   _____

3. mineralization _____

   _____

4. radiologic _____

   _____

5. sciatica _____

   _____

6. tetany _____

   _____

7. tophi _____

   _____

Matching Terms

Match the following terms with the correct definition:

_____ 1. transverse   A. star-like pattern

_____ 2. oblique   B. runs across at a 90-degree angle

_____ 3. spiral   C. twisted around the bone

_____ 4. stellate   D. within the trochanter of the femur

_____ 5. intertrochanteric   E. runs in a transverse pattern

Match the following terms with the correct definition:

____ 6. open fracture

____ 7. simple fracture

____ 8. comminuted

____ 9. stress fracture

____ 10. greenstick

A. more than two ends or fragments

B. bone is protruding through the skin

C. incomplete fracture

D. no opening in the skin

E. too much weight-bearing or pressure

Define Abbreviations

Define the following abbreviations:

1. CAT _____

2. CT _____

3. MRI _____

4. ORIF _____

5. RICE _____

6. LBP _____

7. TMJ _____

8. HNP _____

Identify Diagnostic Tests

Fill in the blanks with the correct terms:

1. The primary tool utilized to diagnose bone and joint disorders is _____.

2. Testing that provides more detail than basic radiologic examination includes _____ and _____.

3. A radiologic examination that provides detailed pictures that appear to cut the area of consideration into slices is _____.

4. A radiologic examination that utilizes a large magnet to make electromagnetic images is _____.

5. _____ studies include calcium, phosphorus, and alkaline phosphatase.

6. Muscle disorders are often evaluated by _____.

Condition Table

Complete the following table:

Condition and Definition	Signs and Symptoms	Diagnostic Tests	Treatment Plan
Scoliosis			
Osteoporosis			
Osteomyelitis			

Osteoarthritis			
Rheumatoid Arthritis			
Muscular Dystrophy			
Fracture			
Herniated Nucleus Pulposus			
Bursitis			
Carpal Tunnel			
Plantar Faciitis			
Cruciate Ligament Tear			

Completion

Using the words in the list, complete the following statements:

kyphosis   scoliosis

lordosis   striated

myelogram   tophi

rickets

1. Muscle that looks like stripes or bands is _____.

2. Small, whitish nodules are called _____.

3. _____ is a humped abnormal curvature of the thoracic spine.

4. Lateral curvature of the spine is called _____.

5. _____ is also called *swayback*.

6. A special X-ray after the injection of dye into the spinal cord to reveal compression of the spinal cord or spinal nerves is called a _____.

Short Answer

Provide answers to the following:

1. What is the difference between cortical bone and cancellous bone?

_____

_____

_____

2. List the steps of bone repair.

   a. _____

   b. _____

   c. _____

   d. _____

   e. _____

3. What factors may affect the healing process?

   a. _____

   b. _____

   c. _____

   d. _____

   e. _____

4. Describe a joint.

   _____

   _____

   _____

5. How are joints classified?

   a. _____

   b. _____

6. List the major movements of the joints.

   a. _____

   b. _____

   c. _____

   d. _____

   e. _____

   f. _____

   g. _____

7. What are the functions of cartilage?

   a. _____

   b. _____

   c. _____

   d. _____

8. What are the functions of muscles?

   a. _____

   b. _____

9. What are tendons?

   _____

   _____

   _____

10. What are common signs and symptoms of bone and joint disease?

    a. _____

    b. _____

    c. _____

    d. _____

11. What are the primary tumors of the bone marrow?

    a. _____

    b. _____

12. What are the most common symptoms of the musculoskeletal system?

    a. _____

    b. _____

13. What are the causes of fractures?

    a. _____

    b. _____

14. Describe the following fractures:

    a. open _____

    b. closed or simple _____

    c. greenstick _____

    d. displaced _____

    e. nondisplaced _____

    f. comminuted _____

    g. compression _____

    h. impacted _____

    i. avulsion _____

    j. longitudinal _____

    k. transverse _____

    l. oblique _____

    m. spiral _____

    n. stellate _____

    o. intracapsular _____

    p. extracapsular _____

    q. intertrochanteric _____

    r. femoral neck/subcapital _____

15. How are fractures treated?

    a. _____

    b. _____

    c. _____

    d. _____

    e. _____

16. What is the benefit of traction when treating fractures?

    a. _____

    b. _____

    c. _____

17. What are two types of traction?

    a. _____

    b. _____

18. What are the complications of fractures?

    a. _____

    b. _____

    c. _____

    d. _____

19. What does the acronym RICE mean?

    R _____

    I _____

    C _____

    E _____

20. What happens to the musculoskeletal system as an individual ages?

    a. _____

    b. _____

    c. _____

    d. _____

    e. _____

    f. _____

True/False

_____ 1. Proper nutrition and calcium are important in reducing risk for osteoporosis.

_____ 2. A shin splint is very similar to a cruciate tear.

_____ 3. Knuckle cracking causes arthritis in the joints.

_____ 4. If you have an injury that has not improved in 7 to 10 days, you should see a physician.

_____ 5. Application of ice on an injury slows bleeding and swelling by causing vasoconstriction.

_____ 6. Spinal manipulation is a frequently prescribed modality for low back pain.

_____ 7. Acupuncture is never used for low back pain because it might do more damage to the spine.

_____ 8. Ice should be applied directly to the skin immediately after an injury.

CASE STUDY

George, age 28, is an avid jogger. He has had some difficulty with shin splints in the past, especially when he has not jogged for a few days and then restarts his exercise routine. He tripped yesterday while jogging and twisted his ankle. He is concerned that he might have sprained it.

1. What are the common symptoms of shin splints?

   _____

   _____

   _____

2. What is the treatment for shin splints?

   _____

   _____

   _____

3. What is a strain?

   _____

   _____

   _____

4. What are the symptoms of a strain?

   _____

   _____

   _____

5. If George has a strain, how should it be treated?

   _____

   _____

6. What is a sprain?

   _____

   _____

   _____

7. What are the symptoms of a sprain?

   _____

   _____

   _____

8. If George has a sprain, how should it be treated?

   _____

   _____

CHAPTER 7

Blood and Blood-Forming Organs Diseases and Disorders

Define Terms

Define the following terms:

1. anemia _____
_____

2. ecchymosis _____
_____

3. erythrocytopenia _____
_____

4. hemarthrosis _____
_____

5. hematemesis _____
_____

6. hematuria _____
_____

7. hemoglobin _____
_____

8. leukocytosis _____
_____

9. pallor _____
_____

10. petechiae _____
_____

11. syncope _____
_____

12. thrombocytosis _____
_____

Matching Terms

Match the following terms with the correct definition:

_____ 1. aplastic anemia

_____ 2. pernicious anemia

_____ 3. hemolytic anemia

_____ 4. sickle cell anemia

_____ 5. hemorrhagic anemia

A. neoplasms of lymphoid tissue

B. failure of bone marrow to produce blood components

C. lack of intrinsic factor

D. acute loss of large amounts of blood

E. increased destruction of red blood cells

F. an inherited anemia

Match the following terms with the correct definition:

_____ 6. hemophilia

_____ 7. pancytopenia

_____ 8. mononucleosis

_____ 9. leukemia

_____ 10. lymphoma

A. decrease in the oxygen-carrying ability of the red blood cell

B. a bleeding disorder; person might need transfusions frequently

C. infection most commonly found in young adults or teens

D. abnormally high number of immature leukocytes

E. malignant neoplasm of blood-forming organs

F. decrease or absence of erythrocytes, leukocytes, and thrombocytes

Define Abbreviations

Define the following abbreviations:

1. RBC _____

2. CBC _____

3. WBC _____

4. Hgb _____

5. Hct _____

Identify Diagnostic Tests

Fill in the blanks with the correct terms:

1. A common blood test that measures the number of RBCs, WBCs, and platelets is called
   a _____.

2. A _____ _____ is a test that provides a detailed count identifying the number of each type of leukocyte.

3. A microscopic examination that identifies the shape of the cells and platelets is a _____ _____.

4. The time it takes for a pricked earlobe to quit bleeding is a test called _____ _____.

5. A test performed by boring a needle into the bone of the iliac crest of the hip to obtain tissue for examination is a _____ _____ _____.

Condition Table

Complete the following table:

Condition and Definition	Signs and Symptoms	Diagnostic Tests	Treatment Plan
Anemia			
Polycythemia			
Leukemia			
Lymphoma			
Multiple Myeloma			
Hemophilia			
Thrombocytopenia			
Disseminated Intravascular Coagulation			
Mononucleosis			

Completion

Using the words in the list, complete the following sentences:

anemia	plasma proteins
hemarthrosis	polycythemia
hematemesis	Reed-Sternberg
hemolyzed	sickle
multiple myeloma	water
pancytopenia	

1. The plasma portion of the blood is composed of _____ and _____ _____.

2. _____ means low or decreased blood volume.

3. An elongated cell with abnormal hemoglobin is called a _____ cell.

4. _____ is an absence or a decrease of erythrocytes, leukocytes, and thrombocytes.

5. Too many blood cells is called _____.

6. A _____ cell is present in the lymphatic tissue in Hodgkin's disease.

7. An excess of calcium may be found in the blood in _____.

8. _____ cells are ones that are broken down.

9. Vomiting blood is also called _____.

10. Bleeding into the joints is called _____.

Short Answer

Provide answers to the following:

1. What is the major function of the blood?

   _____

   _____

   _____

2. What is the role of leukocytes?

   _____

   _____

   _____

3. Describe plasma.

   _____

   _____

   _____

4. What is the function of erythrocytes?

   _____

   _____

   _____

5. What happens to worn-out red blood cells?

   a. _____

   b. _____

6. What is the function of hemoglobin?

   _____

   _____

   _____

7. What is the function of leukocytes?

   _____

   _____

   _____

8. What is the indication of a white blood cell count greater than 11,000?

   _____

   _____

   _____

9. Describe the composition of plasma.

   _____

   _____

   _____

10. List the phases of blood coagulation.

    a. _____

    b. _____

    c. _____

    d. _____

11. List the four types of blood.

    a. _____

    b. _____

    c. _____

    d. _____

12. What is the difference between Rh-negative blood and Rh-positive blood?

    _____

    _____

    _____

13. List the blood-forming organs.

    a. _____

    b. _____

    c. _____

    d. _____

    e. _____

14. What are the common symptoms of erythrocytosis?

    a. _____

    b. _____

    c. _____

    d. _____

    e. _____

15. What happens when an individual has leukocytopenia?

    _____

    _____

    _____

16. What effect does leukocytosis have on the body?

    a. _____

    b. _____

17. What disorders or diseases may lead to anemia?

    a. _____

    b. _____

    c. _____

18. What are the causes of iron deficiency anemia?

    a. _____

    b. _____

19. What are the causes of folic acid deficiency anemia?

    a. _____

    b. _____

    c. _____

    d. _____

20. What race/ethnic group is affected by sickle cell anemia?

    _____

    _____

    _____

21. What is the theory to explain the development of sickle cell anemia?

    _____

    _____

    _____

22. Acute loss of large amounts of blood leads to what type of anemia?

    _____

    _____

    _____

    _____

23. What are the characteristics of aplastic anemia?

    _____

    _____

    _____

24. What are the causes of aplastic anemia?

    a. _____

    b. _____

    c. _____

    d. _____

25. What is the treatment for polycythemia?

    _____

    _____

    _____

26. What are the characteristics of leukemia?

    a. _____

    b. _____

27. What are the characteristics of Hodgkin's disease?

    a. _____

    b. _____

    c. _____

28. What is the cause of Hodgkin's disease?

    _____

    _____

    _____

29. What are the characteristics of thrombocytopenia?

    a. _____

    b. _____

    c. _____

    d. _____

    e. _____

    f. _____

30. When does disseminated intravascular coagulation occur?

    _____

    _____

    _____

31. What is the most common disorder of the blood in the older adult?

    _____

    _____

    _____

True/False

____ 1. Most alternative therapies used to treat leukemia are very effective according to the research.

____ 2. There are many new drugs on the market now for cancer chemotherapy, and many more are being tested and may be available soon.

____ 3. Target-specific drugs are showing promise for treatment regimens for a variety of cancers.

____ 4. The cost versus the need for many other health care interventions for a variety of health issues could lead to fewer new drugs being available for leukemia and other cancers in the future.

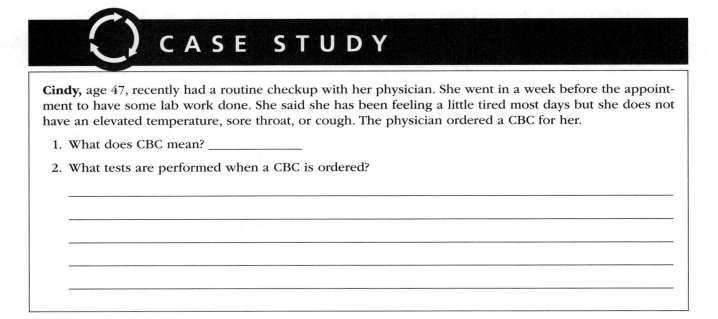

CASE STUDY

Cindy, age 47, recently had a routine checkup with her physician. She went in a week before the appointment to have some lab work done. She said she has been feeling a little tired most days but she does not have an elevated temperature, sore throat, or cough. The physician ordered a CBC for her.

1. What does CBC mean? _____

2. What tests are performed when a CBC is ordered?

   _____

   _____

   _____

   _____

   _____

CHAPTER 8

Cardiovascular System Diseases and Disorders

Define Terms

Define the following terms:

1. auscultation _____

_____

2. cardiac palpitations _____

_____

3. cyanosis _____

_____

4. fibrillation _____

_____

5. ischemia _____

_____

6. murmur _____

_____

7. perfusion _____

_____

8. systolic _____

_____

9. tachycardia _____

_____

10. thrombus _____

_____

Matching Terms

Match the following diagnostic terms with the correct definition:

_____ 1. dyspnea

_____ 2. hemoglobin

_____ 3. arteriogram

_____ 4. ultrasound

_____ 5. angiogram

A. X-ray of an artery

B. carries the oxygen in the blood

C. X-ray of a vessel

D. use of sound waves for diagnostic purposes

E. a device used for listening to the heart and movement of blood in vessels

F. shortness of breath

Match the following diagnostic terms with the correct definition:

_____ 6. patency

_____ 7. Doppler

_____ 8. embolus

_____ 9. prothrombin time

_____ 10. cardiac catheterization

A. material floating in the blood

B. a device that magnifies the sound of blood flow

C. X-ray of an artery

D. invasive procedure used to sample the blood in the chambers of the heart to determine the oxygen content

E. blood test to monitor the anticoagulant drug level

F. openness

Define Abbreviations

Define the following abbreviations:

1. CVA _____

2. EKG or ECG _____

3. MI _____

4. CABG _____

5. CPR _____

6. TPA _____

7. CHF _____

8. DVT _____

Identify Diagnostic Tests

Match the following diagnostic tests with the correct description below:

____ 1. The process of using a stethoscope to listen to the heart

____ 2. A graph picture of heart activity

____ 3. An invasive procedure used to sample the blood in the chambers of the heart to determine the oxygen content and blood pressure in the heart's chambers

____ 4. A device to magnify sounds of the heart and vessels

____ 5. Measured by a sphygmomanometer

____ 6. A blood enzyme indicative of a heart attack

____ 7. A noninvasive ultrasound of the heart

A. cardiac catheterization

B. angiography

C. electrocardiogram

D. venography

E. arterial blood pressure

F. Doppler

G. creatinine phosphokinase

H. echocardiography

I. auscultation

Condition Table

Complete the following table:

Condition and Definition	Signs and Symptoms	Diagnostic Tests	Treatment Plan
Myocardial Infarction			
Hypertensive Heart Disease			
Congestive Heart Failure			
Cardiomyopathy			
Phlebitis			
Varicose Veins			
Hemorrhage			
Shock			

Completion

Using the words in the list, complete the following statements:

arrhythmia	blood pressure	bradycardia
diastolic	dyspnea	embolus
fibrillation	palpitations	plaque
systolic	tachycardia	

1. The top or first recorded number in the blood pressure, caused by the contraction of the ventricle, is the _____ blood pressure.

2. Difficult breathing is also known as _____.

3. _____ _____ is the level of pressure of the blood pushing against the walls of the vessels as it is delivered throughout the body.

4. Fatty, cholesterol deposits in blood vessels are called _____.

5. A blood clot that breaks loose and floats in the blood, possibly occluding or stopping blood flow is known as a(n) _____.

6. An irregular heart rhythm is called a(n) _____.

7. A wild, uncontrolled arrhythmia is called a(n) _____.

8. Another word for rapid heart rate is _____.

9. An abnormal heart rate that the individual can feel or is very aware of is called _____.

10. _____ is a slow heart rate.

11. The bottom number or lower number in the blood pressure is known as the _____ blood pressure.

Short Answer

Describe the following surgical procedures and when they are indicated:

1. Coronary artery bypass graft

   _____
   _____
   _____

2. Endarterectomy

   _____
   _____
   _____

3. Angioplasty

   _____
   _____
   _____

4. Vein stripping

   _____
   _____
   _____

5. Embolectomy/thrombectomy

_____

_____

_____

For each of the following, describe the condition, and then list the symptoms and describe how the disease/disorder is diagnosed:

6. Aneurysm

_____

_____

_____

7. Arteriosclerosis/atherosclerosis

_____

_____

_____

8. Cerebrovascular accident

_____

_____

_____

9. Coronary artery disease

_____

_____

_____

10. Deep vein thrombosis

_____

_____

_____

11. Rheumatic heart disease

_____

_____

_____

_____

12. Peripheral vascular disease

_____

_____

_____

True/False

_____ 1. A recent study noted that weight-loss surgery (bariatric surgery) can reduce the patient's risk of heart attack or stroke.

_____ 2. People with abdominal obesity are more at risk for cardiovascular disease than those who have their weight in the legs and trunk of the body.

_____ 3. It has been proven through research that aromatherapy has no effect on blood pressure.

_____ 4. In the future, people with a high body mass index (BMI) who are recommended for weight-loss surgery might only be those who have abdominal obesity.

_____ 5. There is plenty of evidence that aromatherapy should be used to treat high blood pressure in adults.

_____ 6. An individual needs to have his blood pressure checked routinely only if he has a cardiovascular disease such as hypertension.

↻ CASE STUDY

Evelyn, age 57, is a very active lady in the community. She volunteers at the hospital and also at her church. Lately she had been feeling weak and short of breath and has had some minor chest and leg pains. She has also been having headaches. She knows she is 20 pounds overweight but still has been able to get around fine without any significant trouble. Her physician told her that she has hypertension and some atherosclerosis. She was surprised to hear this because, until recently, she has felt fine. She asked him why she has these problems at this time. He stated that some of this is probably due to heredity but some is related to her lifestyle.

1. The genetic and environmental risk factors contributing to primary hypertension are _____, _____, _____, _____, _____, _____, and _____.

2. The controllable factors contributing to atherosclerosis are _____, _____, _____, _____, _____, _____, and _____.

3. The noncontrollable factors contributing to atherosclerosis are _____, _____, _____, and _____.

CHAPTER 9

Respiratory System Diseases and Disorders

Define Terms

Define the following terms:

1. apnea _____

_____

2. bronchiectasis _____

_____

3. clubbing _____

_____

4. dyspnea _____

_____

5. hemoptysis _____

_____

6. cyanosis _____

_____

7. sputum _____

_____

8. hypoxia _____

_____

9. orthopnea _____

_____

10. tachypnea _____

_____

Matching Terms

Match the disease with the correct identifier:

_____   1. hay fever

_____   2. pharyngitis

_____   3. chronic bronchitis

_____   4. pulmonary abscess

_____   5. tuberculosis

A. sore throat

B. "shock lung"

C. lung abscess

D. worldwide contagious bacterial infection

E. allergic rhinitis

F. obstructive lung disease

Match the following terms with the correct identifier:

_____   6. adult respiratory distress syndrome

_____   7. pleural effusion

_____   8. coccidioidomycosis

_____   9. Legionnaire's disease

_____ 10. laryngitis

A. fungal disease found in desert areas

B. hydrothorax

C. lung membrane inflammation

D. "shock lung"

E. bacterial pneumonia

F. hoarseness

Define Abbreviations

Define the following abbreviations:

1. ABG _____

2. PE _____

3. URI _____

4. TB _____

5. CO_2 _____

6. PFT _____

7. COPD _____

Identify Diagnostic Tests

Match the test with the correct identifier:

_____   1. A group of tests measuring volume and flow of air into the lungs

_____   2. A procedure to look into the lungs

_____   3. The primary or major diagnostic tool

_____   4. A measurement of oxygen and carbon dioxide in the blood

_____   5. A measurement or metered tool to measure lung function

A. auscultation

B. chest roentgenogram

C. bronchoscopy

D. arterial blood gases

E. oxygen saturation

F. pulmonary function tests

G. spirometer

Condition Table

Complete the following table:

Condition and Definition	Signs and Symptoms	Diagnostic Tests	Treatment Plan
Common Cold			
Hay Fever			
Sinusitis			
Pharyngitis			
Acute Bronchitis			
Influenza			
Chronic Obstructive Pulmonary Disease			
Pneumonia			
Tuberculosis			
Pleurisy			
Pulmonary Embolism			
Legionnaire's Disease			
Pneumothorax			

Completion

Using the words in the list, complete the following statements:

orthopnea	rales
rhinorrhea	hypoxia
hemoptysis	dyspnea
antipyretics	apnea
clubbing	analgesics

1. _____ is when an individual is unable to breathe unless the individual is in a sitting position.

2. Musical sounds heard when listening to the lungs are called _____.

3. A runny nose is also called _____.

4. The medical term for low oxygen in the blood is _____.

5. The medical term for coughing up blood is _____.

6. Bad, painful, or difficult breathing is called _____.

7. Medications used to reduce fevers are called _____.

8. Absence of respirations is known as _____.

9. _____ is due to poor distal circulation and oxygenation.

10. Pain relievers are called _____.

Using the words in the list, complete the following statements:

cyanosis	tachypnea
rhonchi	thoracentesis
sputum	wheezing
alveoli	productive cough
bronchoscopy	biopsy

11. A bluish color to the skin is called _____.

12. Rapid breathing is known as _____.

13. Dry, rattling sounds when listening to the lungs are called _____.

14. The surgical puncture of the thorax is known as _____.

15. _____ is fluids or secretions coughed up from the lungs.

16. _____ is a high-pitched whistling sound caused by partial obstruction of the lungs.

17. The grape-like clusters of air sacs at the distal end of the terminal bronchioles are known as _____.

18. A(n) _____ _____ is one in which there is sputum of excessive mucus.

19. The visual examination of the bronchi is called _____.

20. Removing tissue for examination under the microscope is known as a(n) _____.

Using the words in the list, complete the following statements:

hay fever	sinusitis
sore throat	laryngitis
influenza	chronic obstructive pulmonary disease
atelectasis	pneumonia
tuberculosis	lung cancer

21. Allergic rhinitis is commonly known as _____.

22. _____ is inflammation of the mucous membrane lining of the sinuses.

23. Pharyngitis is commonly known as a(n) _____ _____.

24. Inflammation of the vocal cords and larynx is called _____.

25. A highly contagious respiratory infection characterized by sudden onset of fever, chills, headache, and back pain is called _____.

26. A group of diseases characterized by the inability to get air in and out of the lungs is known as _____ _____ _____ _____.

27. Collapse or airless state of part or the entire lung is called _____.

28. Inflammation of the lung is called _____.

29. _____ is an infectious lung problem worldwide.

30. _____ _____ is the leading cause of cancer deaths in the United States.

Using the words in the list, complete the following statements:

pleurisy	pneumothorax
thoracentesis	pleural effusion
pulmonary embolus	histoplasmosis/coccidioidomycosis
smoking	respiratory infection
upper respiratory infections	rhinovirus

31. Inflammation of the membranes covering the lung is called _____.

32. Collection of air in the pleural space is called _____.

33. _____ is a procedure done in order to withdraw air and insert a chest tube to assist in re-expanding the lung.

34. A collection of fluid in the chest is known as _____.

35. A clot that commonly develops in the legs, breaks off, and gets stuck in the pulmonary artery is called a(n) _____ _____.

36. _____ is an example of a fungal disease of the lung.

37. _____ is the most preventable risk factor for developing lung cancer.

38. The type of infection that accounts for approximately 80% of all infections is called _____ _____.

39. The most common cause for lost days of work for adults is _____ _____ _____.

40. The name of the virus responsible for upper respiratory infections is _____.

Short Answer

Provide answers to the following:

1. Describe mechanical ventilation.

   _____

   _____

   _____

2. Describe influenza immunization.

   _____

   _____

   _____

3. Describe a surgical resection of the lung.

   _____

   _____

   _____

4. Describe a salt-water gargle.

_____

_____

_____

True/False

____ 1. Smoking is the main cause of preventable death in the United States.

____ 2. Smoking can cause an increased heart rate.

____ 3. The Centers for Disease Control and Prevention (CDC) recommends using the tuberculosis skin test (TST) for children under age 5.

____ 4. The QuantiFERON-TB (QFT) test is recommended by the CDC for tuberculosis testing particularly for persons who might not return for follow-up.

____ 5. The use of natural immunomodulators (substances that help regulate the immune system, which helps fight infections) has become more popular with the increased acceptance of complementary or alternative therapies.

____ 6. The natural immunomodulators have more side effects than the chemical ones.

CASE STUDY

Joe, age 72, has been diagnosed with pleural effusion. He is having difficulty breathing. The physician said he would need a thoracentesis to relieve the pressure and help his breathing pattern improve.

Describe a thoracentesis procedure.

_____

_____

_____

Lymphatic System Diseases and Disorders

Define Terms

Define the following terms:

1. lymph _____

_____

2. lymphocytes _____

_____

3. lymphocytosis _____

_____

4. lymphocytopenia _____

_____

5. lymphedema _____

_____

Define Terms

Definite the following word forms:

1. lymph _____

_____

2. angio _____

_____

3. adeno _____

_____

4. opathy _____

_____

5. graphy _____

_____

6. itis _____

_____

7. edema _____

_____

8. cyto _____

_____

9. osis _____

_____

10. penia _____

_____

Condition Table

Complete the following table:

Condition and Definition	Signs and Symptoms	Diagnostic Tests	Treatment Plan
Lymphoma			
Kawasaki Disease			
Lymphedema			
Lymphadenitis			

Completion

Using the words in the list, complete the following statements:

Kawasaki disease   lymphocytes
lymph   lymphocytopenia
lymphadenitis   lymphocytosis
lymphadenopathy   lymphomas
lymphangiography   mononucleosis
lymphangiopathy   Reed-Sternberg (RS)
lymphedema   vessels, ducts, nodes

1. Inflammation of the lymph gland and/or nodes is known as _____.

2. Neoplasms that affect lymphoid tissue are called _____.

3. _____ is fluid of the lymph system.

4. White blood cells created in the lymphatic system are called _____.

5. Inflammation of the lymph glands is called _____.

6. An X-ray of the lymph vessels is called _____.

7. A collection of lymph fluid usually in the extremities is called _____.

8. Disease of the lymph vessels is called _____.

9. _____ _____ is also called mucocutaneous lymph node syndrome.

10. _____ is also called the "kissing disease."

11. Decreased lymphocytes are known medically as _____.

12. Increased lymphocytes are medically called _____.

13. Disease of the lymph glands is called _____.

14. The _____ _____ cell confirms the diagnosis of Hodgkin's disease.

15. The lymphatic system includes the _____, _____, and _____.

Short Answer

Provide answers to the following:

1. List the components of the lymph system.

   _____

   _____

   _____

2. What is the goal of the lymphatic system?

   _____

   _____

   _____

3. What is the job of the lymphatic system?

   a._____

   b._____

   c._____

   d._____

   e._____

   f._____

4. List the common signs and symptoms of the lymphatic system.

   a. _____

   b. _____

   c. _____

   d. _____

5. What diagnostic tests are performed in order to confirm a diagnosis of the lymph system?

   a. _____

   b. _____

   c. _____

   d. _____

   e. _____

   f. _____

True/False

_____ 1. Obesity may increase the risk for lymphedema after breast cancer surgery.

_____ 2. Further research needs to be completed to understand why obesity affects lymphedema after breast cancer surgery.

_____ 3. Massage is a common mainstream treatment for lymphedema after breast cancer surgery.

_____ 4. Relaxation therapy is a common alternative treatment used to relieve lymphedema after breast cancer surgery.

_____ 5. Most women with lymphedema after breast cancer surgery have found that alternative treatments to relieve the edema are totally ineffective.

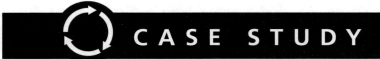

CASE STUDY

Janet, age 19, is a college student. She is not eating or sleeping well, and she recently developed a sore throat. She visited the college health center and was diagnosed with mononucleosis.

1. Describe mononucleosis.

   _____

2. What treatment should she expect?

   _____

CHAPTER 11

Digestive System Diseases and Disorders

Define Terms

Define the following terms:

1. hematochezia _____

   _____

2. diarrhea _____

   _____

3. jejunum _____

   _____

4. achlorhydria _____

   _____

5. defecate _____

   _____

6. epigastric _____

   _____

7. vermiform _____

   _____

8. ileus _____

   _____

9. diverticula _____

   _____

10. asymptomatic _____

    _____

Matching Terms

Match the following terms with the correct definition:

____ 1. an abnormal opening in a tissue or an organ

____ 2. inflammation of the peritoneum

____ 3. contraction of muscles along the gastrointestinal tract to move food

____ 4. vomiting blood

____ 5. tarry, dark stool

A. melena

B. peritonitis

C. peristalsis

D. intrinsic factor

E. hematemesis

F. perforation

Match the following terms with the correct definition:

____ 6. inflammation of the gums

____ 7. parts of tissue that cling to the surface of adjoining organs as scar tissue

____ 8. hidden

____ 9. symptoms flare-up or become worse

____ 10. general ill feeling

A. occult

B. dental plaque

C. malaise

D. adhesions

E. exacerbation

F. gingivitis

Match the following terms with the correct definition:

____ 11. varicose veins in the rectum

____ 12. inflammation of the appendix

____ 13. outpouching of the small intestine and peritoneum into the groin area

____ 14. inflammation of tissue at the lower end of the esophagus

____ 15. inflammation of the stomach and intestine

A. gastroenteritis

B. inguinal hernia

C. hemorrhoids

D. gastritis

E. appendicitis

F. reflux esophagitis

Define Abbreviations

Define the following abbreviations:

1. NPO _____

2. GI _____

3. EGD _____

4. O&P _____

5. IBD _____

6. IBS _____

Identify Diagnostic Tests

Define the following diagnostic tests:

1. colonoscopy _____

2. sigmoidoscopy _____

3. occult blood _____

4. ova and parasites _____

5. upper GI series _____

6. barium enema _____

7. gastroscopy _____

8. esophagogastroduodenoscopy _____

9. stool culture _____

10. biopsy _____

Condition Table

Complete the following table:

Condition and Definition	Signs and Symptoms	Diagnostic Tests	Treatment Plan
Appendicitis			
Reflux Esophagitis			
Pharyngitis			
Crohn's Disease			
Esophageal Varices			
Gastritis			
Peptic Ulcer			
Dysentery			
Colorectal Cancer			
Hemorrhoids			
Inguinal Hernia			
Diverticulitis/Diverticulosis			
Gastroenteritis			

Completion

Using the words in the list, complete the following statements:

duodenum, jejunum, ileum	body
cecum	fundus
intrinsic factor	pylorus
endoscopy	diarrhea
constipation	periodontal disease
sore throat	gingivitis
peristalsis	reflux esophagitis

1. The three sections of the small intestine are the _____, _____, and _____.

2. Movement of food from the pharynx to the stomach is called _____.

3. The first section of the colon is called the _____.

4. The three parts of the stomach are the _____, _____, and _____.

5. The substance necessary for the absorption of vitamin B is called the _____ _____.

6. The condition caused by hard, dry stool is called _____.

7. Loose, watery stools are called _____.

8. The procedure allowing a physician to look directly into the digestive organs is called _____.

9. The main reason for tooth loss is _____ _____.

10. Inflammation of the gums is called _____.

11. The common name for pharyngitis is _____ _____.

12. The backflow of stomach acids through the cardiac sphincter upward into the esophagus is called _____ _____.

Using the words in the list, complete the following statements:

achlorhydria	strangulation
asymptomatic	sprue or celiac disease
pernicious anemia	melena
Crohn's disease	ileus
diverticulitis	hiatal hernia
esophageal varices	hemorrhoids
gastritis	

13. A _____ _____ is the sliding of part of the stomach into the chest cavity.

14. _____ _____ are enlargements of the veins of the esophagus.

15. Inflammation of the stomach is called _____.

16. _____ _____ is the result of the loss of intrinsic factor.

17. Absence of symptoms is also known as _____.

18. _____ is dark, tarry stools.

19. The absence of hydrochloric acid is called _____.

20. Absence of peristalsis is called _____.

21. Varicose veins of the rectum are called _____.

22. When part of the intestine is herniated and becomes twisted, thus cutting off the blood supply to the organ, this is called a _____.

23. Inflammatory bowel syndrome is also called _____ _____.

24. The inflammation of the diverticula is called _____.

25. The condition that causes an individual to be sensitive to gluten proteins is called _____ or _____ _____.

Short Answer

Provide answers to the following:

1. What are the purposes of the digestive system?

   a._____

   b._____

2. Trace a piece of food from the mouth to the anus.

   _____

   _____

3. What are the most common signs and symptoms of gastrointestinal disorders?

   _____

   _____

4. List some causes of constipation.

   _____

   _____

5. List some causes of diarrhea.

   _____

   _____

6. List some effects of aging on the gastrointestinal system.

   _____

   _____

True/False

_____ 1. A low-fiber diet is essential for good GI function.

_____ 2. Continued use of laxative preparations can disrupt the normal GI function.

_____ 3. A strep throat is best diagnosed by inspection.

_____ 4. Antibiotics should be taken as prescribed until all capsules are gone.

_____ 5. Colon cancer is most common before age 40.

_____ 6. Most microorganisms ingested are destroyed by acid in the stomach.

_____ 7. Good hand washing is a preventive strategy for avoiding food poisoning.

_____ 8. The tongue can tell a great deal about the health of a person.

_____ 9. Kudzu root has been used in Chinese herbal medicine for the treatment of several GI disorders.

_____ 10. Chewing and swallowing very rapidly is a good strategy to prevent bloated feelings after eating.

CASE STUDY

Sue is a 36-year-old registered nurse who has been experiencing pain in the epigastric area after eating spicy foods. She has been complaining of the symptoms for the past few weeks.

1. What disease might she have?

   _____

2. How would the diagnosis be made?

   _____

3. How would this disease be treated?

   _____

   _____

   _____

   _____

   _____

   _____

   _____

CHAPTER 12

Liver, Gallbladder, and Pancreatic Diseases and Disorders

Define Terms

Define the following terms:

1. abdominocentesis _____

_____

2. ascites _____

_____

3. cholecystectomy _____

_____

4. esophageal varices _____

_____

5. hematemesis _____

_____

6. hepatomegaly _____

_____

7. jaundice _____

_____

8. splenomegaly _____

_____

Matching Terms

Match the following terms with the correct definition:

_____ 1. a yellow skin color related to bile pigments in the blood

_____ 2. occurring suddenly, rapidly, and intensely

_____ 3. digestion of self or one's own cells

_____ 4. fluid in the abdomen

_____ 5. a serious condition due to alcohol withdrawal

A. jaundice

B. ascites

C. autodigestion

D. delirium tremens

E. fulminant

F. gynecomastia

Identify Diagnostic Tests

Match the following diagnostic tests with the correct definition:

_____ 1. cholecystogram

_____ 2. amylase

_____ 3. needle biopsy

_____ 4. alkaline phosphatase

_____ 5. albumin

_____ 6. cholangiogram

_____ 7. abdominocentesis

_____ 8. lithotripsy

_____ 9. liver function tests

_____ 10. ultrasound

A. blood protein

B. X-ray of the gallbladder

C. evaluates the liver, gallbladder, and pancreas for size, shape, and position

D. surgical puncture of abdomen

E. measures pancreatic function

F. enzyme

G. sound waves used to break up stones

H. measures levels of bilirubin, albumin, and alkaline phosphatase

I. X-ray of the vessels of the gallbladder

J. most reliable test for diagnosis of cancer, chronic hepatitis, and cirrhosis

Condition Table

Complete the following table:

Condition and Definition	Signs and Symptoms	Diagnostic Tests	Treatment Plan
Cirrhosis			
Hepatitis B			
Cholecystitis			
Cholelithiasis			
Pancreatitis			

Completion

Using the words in the list, complete the following statements:

autodigestion	jaundice
cholelithiasis	hyperbilirubinemia
lithotripsy	emesis
ascites	hematemesis

1. Digestion of one's own cells is called _____.

2. The yellowish discoloration of the skin is known as _____.

3. The medical term for gallstones is _____.

4. Excessive bilirubin in the blood is called _____.

5. The use of sound waves to break up gallstones is called _____.

6. Vomiting is also called _____.

7. _____ is the accumulation of fluid in the abdomen.

8. Vomiting blood is also called _____.

Using the words in the list, complete the following statements:

abdominocentesis	spider angiomas
cholangiogram	pancreatitis
cholecystitis	liver
cholecystogram	hepatomegaly
hepatitis	fulminant

9. _____ is an enlarged liver.

10. Small dilated blood vessels on the face and chest are called _____ _____.

11. _____ is puncture of the abdomen.

12. A _____ is an X-ray of the gallbladder.

13. Inflammation of the liver is commonly called _____.

14. _____ is when something occurs suddenly and with great intensity.

15. The _____ is the largest solid organ of the body.

16. Inflammation of the gallbladder is called _____.

17. X-ray of the vessels of the gallbladder is called _____.

Short Answer

Provide answers to the following:

1. Describe the functions of the liver.

   a. _____

   b. _____

   c. _____

d. _____

e. _____

f. _____

g. _____

h. _____

i. _____

2. Identify two signs and/or symptoms of liver problems.

_____

_____

_____

3. Describe bile and its function.

_____

_____

_____

4. The pancreas is both an endocrine and an exocrine gland. What does this mean?

_____

_____

_____

5. What are the secretions of the pancreas?

_____

_____

_____

6. Older adults may be at risk for pancreatitis if what factors are present?

a. _____

b. _____

c. _____

d. _____

e. _____

f. _____

True/False

_____ 1. Good elimination habits include a high-fiber diet, daily exercise, and adequate fluid intake.

_____ 2. The mortality rate of hepatitis increases with age.

_____ 3. Chronic hepatitis C is a regional disease but not a health threat worldwide.

_____ 4. In studies of the Chinese herbal medicine Sho-saiko-to, it was found that the herb product was not at all effective for preventing cancer in patients with cirrhosis.

CASE STUDY

Jean is 45 years old and 50 pounds overweight. For the past 3 weeks, Jean has been experiencing severe right upper gastric pain after eating. She is diagnosed with cholecystitis.

1. What is this disease?

   _____

   _____

2. What predisposing factors does she have?

   _____

   _____

3. What symptoms does she have to support the diagnosis?

   _____

   _____

4. How would the diagnosis be confirmed?

   _____

   _____

5. What treatment might be done?

   _____

   _____

   _____

CHAPTER 13

Urinary System Diseases and Disorders

Define Terms

Define the following terms:

1. anuria _____

   _____

2. catheterization _____

   _____

3. cystoscopy _____

   _____

4. dysuria _____

   _____

5. hematuria _____

   _____

6. nephrectomy _____

   _____

7. nocturia _____

   _____

8. uremia _____

   _____

9. pyuria _____

   _____

10. suprapubic catheter _____

    _____

Matching Terms

Match the following terms with the correct definition:

____ 1. collection of urine in the renal pelvis due to obstruction

____ 2. any infection of the urinary system

____ 3. kidney stones

____ 4. inflammation of the bladder

____ 5. painful urination

A. hydronephrosis

B. urinary tract infection

C. renal calculi

D. glomerulonephritis

E. cystitis

F. dysuria

Match the following terms with the correct definition:

____ 6. multiple grape-like cysts

____ 7. failure of the kidneys to perform the function of cleansing the blood of waste products

____ 8. urine waste in the blood

____ 9. inflammation of the urethra

____ 10. excision of a kidney

A. pyelonephritis

B. renal failure

C. polycystic disease

D. uremia

E. urethritis

F. nephrectomy

Define Abbreviations

Define the following abbreviations:

1. KUB _____

2. TUR _____

3. IVP _____

4. BUN _____

5. C&S _____

6. UTI _____

Identify Diagnostic Tests

Match the following diagnostic tests with the correct definition:

____ 1. clean catch

____ 2. urine C&S

____ 3. needle biopsy

____ 4. blood urea nitrogen

____ 5. creatinine clearance

____ 6. urinalysis

____ 7. KUB

____ 8. lithotripsy

____ 9. catheterization

____ 10. cystoscopy

A. the most common test to diagnose urinary system diseases

B. X-ray examination of kidney, ureters and bladder

C. obtaining clean urine for culture

D. breaking up kidney stones

E. a blood test to measure kidney function

F. lab test used if urine shows abnormal WBC or bacteria

G. protein waste in the blood

H. obtaining a small piece of tissue to determine the presence of disease

I. sterile procedure of placing a tube in the bladder

J. looking into the bladder

Condition Table

Complete the following table:

Condition and Definition	Signs and Symptoms	Diagnostic Tests	Treatment Plan
Polycystic Disease			
Renal Failure			
Glomerulonephritis			
Cystitis			
Pyelonephritis			
Transitional Cell Carcinoma of the Bladder			
Hydronephrosis			

Completion

Using the words in the list, complete the following statements:

anuria

cystitis

cystoscopy

dysuria

hematuria

incontinence

nocturia

oliguria

pyretic

pyuria

renal calculi

urgency

1. Inflammation of the bladder is called _____.

2. Another term for having a fever is _____.

3. Kidney stones are also called _____ _____.

4. _____ is blood in the urine.

5. The need to urinate "right now" is called _____.

6. _____ is loss of control of urine.

7. The need to urinate at night is called _____.

8. Bad, painful, or difficult urination is called _____.

9. Scant urine production is called _____.

10. Visual examination of the bladder is called _____.

11. Absence of urine is called _____.

12. Pus in the urine is called _____.

Short Answer

Provide answers to the following:

1. Describe the anatomy of the urinary system.

   _____

   _____

   _____

   _____

2. What signs and symptoms are commonly seen in urinary system disorders?

   _____

   _____

   _____

3. What is the function of the kidney?

   _____

   _____

   _____

4. Describe urine.

   _____

   _____

   _____

True/False

_____   1. Limiting fluid intake might prevent recurring urinary tract infections.

_____   2. Drinking cranberry juice is recommended to raise the pH of the urine to prevent infections.

_____   3. Eating large amounts of red meat may increase one's risk of developing kidney cancer.

_____   4. Research has found that *Palicourea* (an herbal medicine) does act as a diuretic.

_____   5. More research is needed to determine the effectiveness of *Palicourea coriacea* K. Schum for treatment of kidney disease.

_____   6. There is no link between eating grilled red meat and kidney cancer.

_____   7. Red meat of any kind in any amount has not been found to be harmful to one's health.

_____   8. Federal guidelines suggest that all people should eat lean meat, fish, and poultry.

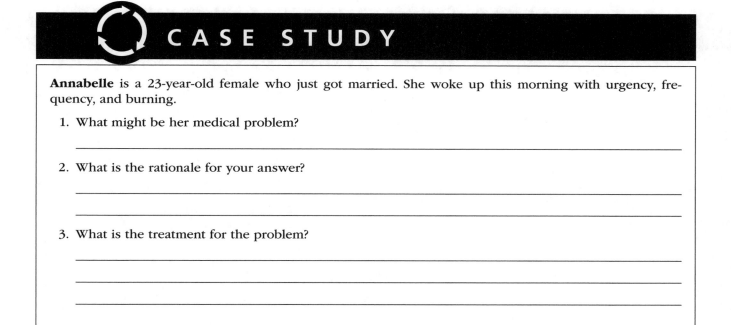

CASE STUDY

Annabelle is a 23-year-old female who just got married. She woke up this morning with urgency, frequency, and burning.

1. What might be her medical problem?

   _____

2. What is the rationale for your answer?

   _____

   _____

3. What is the treatment for the problem?

   _____

   _____

   _____

CHAPTER 14

Endocrine System Diseases and Disorders

Define Terms

Define the following terms:

1. adenoma _____
   _____

2. androgen _____
   _____

3. glucagon _____

4. hirsutism _____
   _____

5. islets of Langerhans _____
   _____

6. polyuria _____
   _____

7. precocious _____
   _____

8. striae _____
   _____

9. tetany _____
   _____

10. vasopressin _____
    _____

Matching Terms

Match the following terms with the correct definition:

_____ 1. hyperpituitarism

_____ 2. type 1 diabetes

_____ 3. cretinism

_____ 4. Graves' disease

_____ 5. diabetes insipidus

A. formerly known as juvenile onset diabetes

B. decrease in the release of vasopressin

C. abnormal increase in the activity of the pituitary gland

D. hypothyroidism in infants and children

E. formerly known as adult onset diabetes

F. hyperthyroidism caused by an autoimmune disorder

Match the following terms with the correct definition:

_____ 6. goiter

_____ 7. Cushing's syndrome

_____ 8. polydipsia

_____ 9. Addison's disease

_____ 10. type 2 diabetes

A. enlargement of the thyroid gland due to inadequate dietary iodine

B. formerly known as adult-onset diabetes

C. overproduction of cortisone

D. overproduction of aldosterone

E. hypoadrenalism

F. excessive thirst or drinking

Define Abbreviations

Match the following abbreviations with the correct definition:

_____ 1. TSH

_____ 2. FSH

_____ 3. GH

_____ 4. ADH

_____ 5. MSH

_____ 6. ACTH

_____ 7. LH

_____ 8. ICSH

_____ 9. IDDM

_____ 10. STH

A. somatropin hormone

B. antidiuretic hormone

C. non–insulin-dependent diabetes mellitus

D. follicle-stimulating hormone

E. growth hormone

F. interstitial cell–stimulating hormone

G. adrenocorticotropin hormone

H. insulin-dependent diabetes mellitus

I. thyroid-stimulating hormone

J. luteinizing hormone

K. melanocyte-stimulating hormone

Identify Diagnostic Tests

Mark an "X" in front of the basic diagnostic tests used to diagnose endocrine disorders:

A. _____ CT

B. _____ MRI

C. _____ Electrocardiogram

D. _____ Physical examination

E. _____ Blood tests

F. _____ Esophagogastroduodenoscopy

G. _____ Colonoscopy

H. _____ Upper GI

Define Word Forms

Define the following word forms:

1. dipsia _____

2. poly _____

3. anti _____

4. uri _____

5. oma _____

6. glyc _____

7. phagia _____

8. adeno _____

9. hyper _____

10. hypo _____

Condition Table

Complete the following table:

Condition and Definition	Signs and Symptoms	Diagnostic Tests	Treatment Plan
Goiter			
Diabetes Mellitus			
Diabetes Insipidus			
Giantism			
Addison's Disease			
Hypothyroidism			
Hypogonadism			
Conn's Disease			
Hyperparathyroidism			

Completion

Using the words in the list, complete the following statements:

growth hormone	gigantism
dwarfism	diabetes insipidus
thyroxine	Graves' disease
thyroid storm	goiter
cretinism	hypoparathyroidism

1. _____ _____ promotes the growth and development of all body tissues.

2. Hyperpituitarism occurring before puberty is known as _____.

3. Hypopituitarism results in _____.

4. A decrease in the release of vasopressin results in _____.

5. The hormone _____ regulates metabolism.

6. Hyperthyroidism caused by an autoimmune condition is also known as _____.

7. _____ _____ is a life-threatening exacerbation of all symptoms of hyperthyroidism.

8. An enlargement of the thyroid gland due to inadequate dietary iodine is called _____.

9. Hypothyroidism in children is called _____.

10. Low blood calcium levels result in _____.

Using the words in the list, complete the following statements:

Addison's disease	Cushing's disease
diabetic coma	gestational diabetes
hypogonadism	insulin, glucagon
insulin shock	ketoacidosis
ketones	polydipsia, polyphagia, polyuria

11. _____ _____ is due to an overproduction of cortisol.

12. Undersecretion of hormones produced by the adrenal cortex is called _____ _____.

13. The two hormones secreted by the pancreas are _____ and _____.

14. When cells burn fats and proteins for energy, they produce a waste product called _____.

15. The condition of having ketones in the blood, breath, and urine is called _____.

16. Three symptoms of diabetes mellitus include _____, _____, and _____.

17. A condition that comes on rapidly as a result of too much insulin is called _____ _____.

18. _____ _____ is the result of not administering enough insulin or taking in too many carbohydrates in the diet.

19. _____ _____ is a result of pregnancy.

20. Decreased production of sex hormones results in _____.

Short Answer

Provide answers to the following:

1. Describe the components of the endocrine system and their location.

   a. _____

   b. _____

   c. _____

   d. _____

   e. _____

   f. _____

   g. _____

   h. _____

   i. _____

2. List some common signs and symptoms of endocrine system disorders.

_____

_____

_____

3. List the endocrine glands and their hormones.

a. _____

b. _____

c. _____

d. _____

e. _____

f. _____

g. _____

h. _____

i. _____

4. List the symptoms of insulin shock.

_____

_____

5. List the symptoms of diabetic coma.

_____

_____

True/False

____ 1. The American Diabetes Association (ADA) recommends that individuals be checked for diabetes every 3 years after age 45.

____ 2. In assessing for diabetes risk, body mass index (BMI) is not important to determine.

____ 3. There is a "Changing Health Habits Assessment" on the ADA Web site that individuals can review for help in lowering the risk for diabetes.

____ 4. A link has been found between the use of statins and diabetes in older women.

____ 5. New research has shown that a person would have to drink only one cup of black tea per week to reduce the risk for diabetes.

____ 6. There are no complementary or alternative strategies for reducing one's risk for diabetes.

____ 7. Health care providers should monitor older women who are taking statins for early signs of diabetes.

____ 8. New research has reported that black tea may reduce an individual's risk for diabetes.

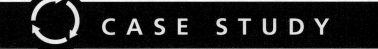

CASE STUDY

Lydia is a 50-year-old businesswoman who has noticed a slight enlargement in her neck. Her mother had a goiter at about the same age Lydia is now, so she is concerned that she may also have a goiter. She knows a goiter merely means enlargement of the thyroid gland.

What symptoms might Lydia exhibit if the goiter is due to hyperthyroidism?

_____

_____

_____

CHAPTER 15

Nervous System Diseases and Disorders

Define Terms

Define the following terms:

1. intractable _____

   _____

2. paresthesia _____

   _____

3. quadriplegia _____

   _____

4. cephalalgia _____

   _____

5. sleep apnea _____

   _____

6. amnesia _____

   _____

7. hypothermia _____

   _____

8. insomnia _____

   _____

9. seizure _____

   _____

10. hydrophobia _____

    _____

Matching Terms

Match the following terms with the correct definition:

_____   1. nuchal rigidity

_____   2. transient ischemic attacks

_____   3. spinal stenosis

_____   4. craniotomy

_____   5. paraplegia

A. sudden, mild "mini strokes"

B. loss of movement in both legs

C. neck stiffness

D. narrowing of nerve root openings

E. loss of movement in all extremities

F. cutting into the skull

Match the following terms with the correct definition:

_____   6. aura

_____   7. dementia

_____   8. endarterectomy

_____   9. decompression

_____ 10. obstructive apnea

A. loss of mental ability

B. release pressure off the spinal cord

C. cleaning plaque out of an artery

D. fear of water

E. not breathing related to nasal blocking

F. sensation that precedes an event

Define Abbreviations

Define the following abbreviations:

1. CSF _____

2. TIA _____

3. CVA _____

4. HNP _____

5. EEG _____

Identify Diagnostic Tests

Define the following diagnostic tests:

1. spinal tap/lumbar puncture _____

2. electroencephalogram _____

3. motor testing _____

4. sensory testing _____

5. mental or cognitive testing _____

6. cerebrospinal fluid analysis _____

7. myelogram _____

8. angiograms _____

Condition Table

Complete the following table:

Condition and Definition	Signs and Symptoms	Diagnostic Tests	Treatment Plan
Parkinson's Disease			
Concussion/Contusion			
Subdural Hematoma			
Meningitis			
Encephalitis			
Shingles			
Cerebrovascular Accident			
Transient Ischemic Attacks			
Headaches			
Epilepsy			
Bell's Palsy			
Alzheimer's Disease			
Sleep Apnea			

Completion

Using the words in the list, complete the following statements:

cephalalgia	convulsions
intractable	transient ischemic attacks
sleep apnea	insomnia
concussion	amnesia
craniotomy	hydrophobia

1. _____ is another name for headaches.

2. Abnormal muscle contractions are known as _____.

3. _____ means difficult to stop or control.

4. _____ _____ _____ are also called "mini strokes."

5. _____ _____ means without sleep.

6. The inability to fall or stay asleep is called _____.

7. A blow to the head by an object, fall, or other trauma is known as a(n) _____.

8. _____ is loss of memory.

9. An incision into the skull is called _____.

10. _____ is throat spasms caused by the sight of water or attempting to drink water.

Using the words in the list, complete the following statements:

status epilepticus	paresthesia
quadriplegia	encephalitis
pia mater	nuchal rigidity
paraplegia	Parkinson's disease
dura mater, arachnoid, pia mater	central

11. Constant jerky uncontrollable movement is called _____ _____.

12. _____ is an abnormal sensation, burning, tingling, or numbness.

13. Paralysis of all four extremities is called _____.

14. Inflammation of the brain is called _____.

15. _____ _____ is the inner layer of the meninges.

16. _____ _____ is a condition where the neck resists bending forward or sideways.

17. Paralysis below the waist is called _____.

18. Pill-rolling of the fingers is a classic symptom of _____.

19. The brain and the spinal cord make up the _____ nervous system.

20. The three layers of the meninges are called the _____, _____, and _____.

Using the words in the list, complete the following statements:

amyotrophic lateral sclerosis	Bell's palsy
electroencephalogram	epilepsy
headaches	multiple sclerosis
shingles	sleep apnea
spinal fluid	status epilepticus

21. The circulating fluid in the brain and spinal cord is called _____ _____.

22. A(n) _____ is a procedure to evaluate electrical brain activity.

23. _____ is a disease caused by the virus herpes zoster.

24. Tension, cluster, and migraine are types of _____.

25. A chronic disease of the brain characterized by intermittent episodes of abnormal electrical activity is called _____.

26. _____ _____ is a state of continued convulsive seizure with no recovery of consciousness.

27. A disease causing unilateral paralysis of the face is called _____ _____.

28. A sleep disorder characterized by periods of apnea or breathlessness is called _____ _____.

29. Demyelination of the nerves of the central nervous system is called _____ _____.

30. A destructive disease of the motor neurons is called _____ _____ _____.

Short Answer

Provide answers to the following:

1. Describe the components of the nervous system.

   _____

   _____

   _____

2. What are the common signs and symptoms of nervous system disorders?

   a. _____

   b. _____

   c. _____

3. List the cranial nerves and their function(s).

   a. _____

   b. _____

   c. _____

   d. _____

   e. _____

   f. _____

   g. _____

   h. _____

   i. _____

   j. _____

   k. _____

   l. _____

4. Describe the spinal nerves.

   _____

   _____

   _____

True/False

_____ 1. There are three distinct polioviruses designated as types 1, 2, and 3.

_____ 2. Dr. Jonas Salk developed an oral vaccine against all three forms of virus called a trivalent vaccine (TOPV—trivalent oral polio vaccine).

_____ 3. Many individuals today are taking mega-doses of vitamins for a variety of reasons.

_____ 4. A group of doctors and researchers warn the consumer that taking large doses of vitamins might actually be harmful to their health.

_____ 5. Large amounts of vitamin D and calcium with large amounts of vitamin E are necessary to reduce a person's risk of hemorrhagic stroke by 22%.

_____ 6. Your diet has nothing to do with your ability to think well when taking tests.

_____ 7. Diets high in vitamins and omega-3 fatty acids are good for brain health.

_____ 8. Recent research found that patients with Parkinson's disease who took a combination of herbs, which included *gou teng*, were able to sleep well and had more understandable speech patterns.

CASE STUDY

Joseph is an 80-year-old grandfather of six children. The ages of his grandchildren range from 11 to 35. At a recent family reunion, several of them stated concern about their grandfather's decreasing functioning. They were told this is a typical occurrence in aging.

What are the normal effects of aging on the nervous system?

_____

_____

_____

CHAPTER 16

Eye and Ear Diseases and Disorders

Define Terms

Define the following terms:

1. cerumen _____
   _____

2. diplopia _____
   _____

3. ophthalmoscope _____
   _____

4. otoscope _____
   _____

5. otalgia _____
   _____

6. tonometry _____
   _____

7. stapedectomy _____
   _____

8. vertigo _____
   _____

9. myringotomy _____
   _____

10. pruritus _____
    _____

Matching Terms

Match the following terms with the correct definition:

____ 1. amblyopia

____ 2. enucleation

____ 3. mastoidectomy

____ 4. photophobia

____ 5. pruritus

A. itching

B. fear of light

C. removal of the eyeball

D. caused by a pathogen or a disease

E. removal of the mastoid bone

F. decrease in vision due to lack of stimuli

Match the following terms with the correct definition:

____ 6. suppurative

____ 7. tinnitus

____ 8. topical

____ 9. tympanoplasty

____ 10. purulent

A. placed on the skin

B. formation of pus

C. surgical repair of the eardrum

D. ringing in the ears

E. referring to the entire body

F. full of dead neutrophils and bacteria

Identify Diagnostic Tests

Explain the following tests:

1. ophthalmoscopy _____

2. visual acuity measurement _____

3. tonometry _____

4. slit-lamp examination _____

5. angiography _____

6. otoscopic examination _____

7. audiometry _____

Condition Table

Complete the following table:

Condition and Definition	Signs and Symptoms	Diagnostic Tests	Treatment Plan
Retinal Detachment			
Otosclerosis			
Diabetic Retinopathy			
Mastoiditis			

Otitis Media			
Ménière's Disease			
Cataracts			
Strabismus			
Macular Degeneration			

Completion

Using the words in the list, complete the following statements:

anterior chamber	pinna
choroid layer	pupil
cornea	retina
iris	sclera
lens	tympanic membrane

1. _____ is also known as the outer ear.

2. The clear fibers enclosed in a membrane that refract and focus light to the retina are called the _____.

3. _____ _____ is also known as the eardrum.

4. The clear tissue that covers the pupil and iris is called the _____.

5. _____ is the inside layer of the posterior part of the eye that receives light rays.

6. The layer between the sclera and the retina containing blood vessels is called the _____ _____.

7. _____ is the round disk of muscles that gives the eye its color.

8. The white area covering the outside of the eye except over the pupil and iris is called the _____ _____.

9. _____ is the round opening in the iris that changes its size as the iris reacts to light and dark.

10. The space between the cornea and the iris is called the _____ _____.

Short Answer

Provide answers to the following:

1. List the anatomical components of the eyes.

   a. extraocular

   1. _____

   2. _____

   3. _____

4. _____

5. _____

b. intraocular

1. _____

2. _____

3. _____

4. _____

5. _____

6. _____

7. _____

8. _____

9. _____

10. _____

11. _____

2. List the anatomical components of the ear.

_____

_____

_____

3. Which cranial nerves innervate the eye?

a. _____

b. _____

c. _____

d. _____

e. _____

f. _____

4. How are sound waves transferred to the brain?

_____

_____

_____

_____

5. How does the ear help the body maintain equilibrium?

_____

_____

_____

6. What are some common signs and symptoms of eye disorders?

_____

_____

_____

7. What are some common signs and symptoms of ear disorders?

_____

_____

_____

True/False

_____ 1. Eye strain and fatigue associated with sitting long hours in front of a computer is now called computer vision syndrome.

_____ 2. Research has shown that carotenoid antioxidants increase blood flow and reduce eye irritation and inflammation.

_____ 3. A new vitamin formula specifically targeting eye strain and eye fatigue has yet to be developed, but one is in the process of being researched.

_____ 4. There are several new drugs on the market to treat age-related macular degeneration, and the Food and Drug Administration recently approved an implantable miniature telescope.

_____ 5. Placement of bilateral cochlear implants has improved the quality of life of those receiving them.

_____ 6. Children who are deaf who have had cochlear implants have reported a significant improvement in quality of life.

_____ 7. Arcus senilis rarely occurs in the older adult.

_____ 8. Age-related macular degeneration (AMD) is the leading cause of severe vision loss and blindness in the older adult.

CASE STUDY

Lilly is a 67-year-old retired teacher. She has noticed blurring and decreasing vision over the past few months. She visited her ophthalmologist, who diagnosed her with cataracts. She is concerned about the condition of her eyes and eventual treatment of the cataracts.

What is the expected treatment for Lilly's condition?

_____

_____

_____

CHAPTER 17

Reproductive System Diseases and Disorders

Define Terms

Define the following terms:

1. amenorrhea _____
   _____

2. leukorrhea _____
   _____

3. chancre _____
   _____

4. epididymitis _____
   _____

5. septicemia _____
   _____

6. vaginitis _____
   _____

7. prophylactic _____
   _____

8. ectopic _____
   _____

9. primigravid _____
   _____

10. antiemetic _____
    _____

Matching Terms

Match the following terms with the correct definition:

_____ 1. prepuce

_____ 2. dysmenorrhea

_____ 3. menorrhagia

_____ 4. metrorrhagia

_____ 5. dyspareunia

A. state of being inactive

B. painful menses

C. excessive menses

D. excessive bleeding between menstrual periods

E. painful sexual intercourse

F. foreskin

Match the following terms with the correct definition:

_____ 6. leiomyomas

_____ 7. multiparity

_____ 8. proteinuria

_____ 9. uterine prolapse

_____ 10. mammoplasty

A. surgical reconstruction of the breasts

B. uterus drops or protrudes downward

C. protein or albumin in the urine

D. multiple births

E. benign tumors of the uterus

F. white vaginal discharge

Define Abbreviations

Define the following abbreviations:

1. VDRL _____

2. D&C _____

3. PID _____

4. PMS _____

5. BPH _____

6. STD _____

7. AIDS _____

8. TURP _____

Identify Diagnostic Tests

Define the following diagnostic tests:

1. laparoscopy _____

2. hysterosalpingogram _____

3. bimanual examination _____

4. cytologic _____

5. mammogram _____

6. digital rectal examination _____

7. Pap smear _____

8. culture and sensitivity _____

9. prostate-specific antigen _____

Condition Table

Complete the following table:

Disease Condition and Definition	Signs and Symptoms	Diagnostic Tests	Treatment Plan
Benign Prostatic Hyperplasia			
Ectopic Pregnancy			
Hyperemesis Gravidarum			
Abruptio Placentae			
Placenta Previa			
Toxic Shock Syndrome			
Menopause			
Mastectomy			
Premenstrual Syndrome			
Endometriosis			

Completion

Using the words in the list, complete the following statements:

amenorrhea
dyspareunia
dysmenorrhea
hysterosalpingogram
cytology
spontaneous abortion

endometriosis
metrorrhagia
menorrhagia
laparoscopy
prepuce
hyperemesis

1. _____ means without menses.

2. Abnormal growth of the lining of the uterus outside the uterus is called _____.

3. _____ is painful sexual intercourse.

4. Abnormal bleeding between menstrual periods is called _____.

5. Bad, painful, or difficult menses is known as _____.

6. _____ is excessive or prolonged menstrual bleeding.

7. An X-ray of the uterus and the fallopian tubes is called a(n) _____.

8. A procedure done to look inside the abdominal cavity is called a(n) _____.

9. The study of cells is called _____.

10. The medical term for the foreskin is _____.

11. _____ _____ is commonly known as a miscarriage.

12. _____ is excessive vomiting.

Using the words in the list, complete the following statements:

chancre	digital rectal examination
syphilis	menopause
mastectomy	cervicitis
clap	cryptorchidism
ectopic pregnancy	epididymitis
hysterosalpingogram	orchidectomy
preeclampsia	primigravida

13. Another name for toxemia is _____.

14. The medical term for first pregnancy is _____.

15. A pregnancy that occurs when the fertilized ovum attaches outside the uterus is called _____.

16. Surgical excision of the testes is called a(n) _____.

17. _____ is undescended testicles.

18. Inflammation of the storage tank for sperm is called _____.

19. The slang word for gonorrhea is _____.

20. A painless, highly contagious lesion is called _____.

21. In order to feel the prostate, the physician must perform a _____ _____ _____.

22. A VDRL and an RPR are blood tests performed to test for _____.

23. The natural halting of menstruation is called _____.

24. The surgical excision of the breast is called _____.

25. Inflammation of the cervix is called _____.

Short Answer

Provide answers to the following:

1. List the components of the reproductive system.

   Female:

   _____

   _____

   _____

   _____

Male:

_____

_____

_____

_____

2. What are the common signs and symptoms of reproductive system disorders?

Female:

_____

_____

_____

_____

Male:

_____

_____

_____

_____

3. Explain the following procedures:

a. lumpectomy _____

b. mastectomy _____

c. mammoplasty _____

d. panhysterectomy _____

e. orchiectomy _____

f. transurethral resection of the prostate _____

g. A&P repair _____

h. cystoscopy _____

i. hysterectomy _____

j. D&C _____

True/False

____ 1. A recent study on women's health found that coffee drinkers had less depression than those who did not drink coffee.

____ 2. Coffee usually contains about twice as much caffeine per cup as tea.

____ 3. New research has shown that weightlifting increases the symptoms in women who have not yet developed lymphedema after breast cancer surgery.

____ 4. It is possible to be infected with a sexually transmitted infection without knowing it.

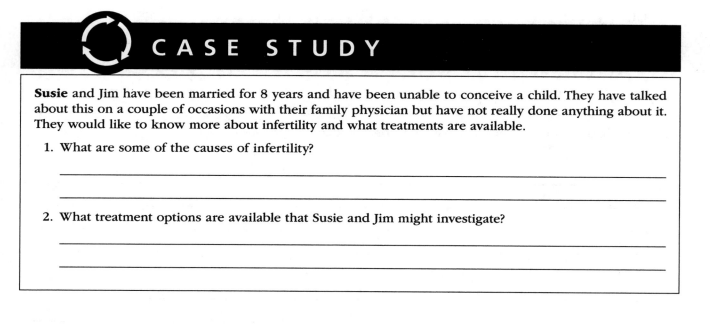

CASE STUDY

Susie and Jim have been married for 8 years and have been unable to conceive a child. They have talked about this on a couple of occasions with their family physician but have not really done anything about it. They would like to know more about infertility and what treatments are available.

1. What are some of the causes of infertility?

   _____

   _____

2. What treatment options are available that Susie and Jim might investigate?

   _____

   _____

CHAPTER 18

Integumentary System Diseases and Disorders

Define Terms

Define the following terms:

1. abrasion _____

   _____

2. comedones _____

   _____

3. erythema _____

   _____

4. lesion _____

   _____

5. pruritus _____

   _____

6. sebum _____

   _____

7. vesicles _____

   _____

8. pustules _____

   _____

9. keratin _____

   _____

10. ulcer _____

    _____

Matching Terms

Match the disease with the correct definition:

_____ 1. seborrheic dermatitis of an infant

_____ 2. eczema

_____ 3. scleroderma

_____ 4. erysipelas

_____ 5. pediculosis

_____ 6. scabies

_____ 7. tinea pedis

_____ 8. folliculitis

_____ 9. herpes varicella

_____ 10. herpes zoster

A. a contagious infection of the skin caused by a mite

B. shingles

C. cellulitis of the dermis caused by group A *Streptococcus*

D. chickenpox

E. atopic dermatitis

F. inflammation and infection of the hair follicle

G. hardening of the skin

H. athlete's foot

I. lice

J. "cradle cap"

Identify Diagnostic Tests

Define the following diagnostic tests:

1. culture and sensitivity _____

2. skin scrapings _____

3. incision and drainage (I&D) _____

4. curettage _____

5. biopsy _____

Condition Table

Complete the following table:

Condition and Definition	Signs and Symptoms	Diagnostic Tests	Treatment Plan
Herpes			
Impetigo			
Abscess, Furuncle, and Carbuncle			
Lyme Disease			
Tinea Pedis			
Candidiasis			

Pediculosis			
Acne			
Seborrheic Dermatitis			
Eczema			
Psoriasis			
Malignant Melanoma			
Burns: First-, Second-, and Third-Degree			
Pressure (Decubitus) Ulcer			
Corns and Calluses			
Ringworm			

Completion

Using the words in the list, complete the following statements:

abrasion	pilonidal cyst
comedone	pruritus
erythema	pustule
lesion	sebum
paronychia	ulcer
papule	wheal

1. _____ is produced by the sebaceous glands.

2. _____ is the medical term for redness.

3. Severe itching is also known as _____.

4. A broad term meaning abnormality of tissue or any discontinuity is called a(n) _____.

5. A(n) _____ is a small circumscribed elevation of the skin containing pus.

6. A small solid raised lesion less than 0.5 cm in diameter is called a(n) _____.

7. A(n) _____ is an open sore or erosion of the skin or mucous membrane.

8. A smooth, slightly elevated, swollen area that is redder or paler than the surrounding skin and is usually accompanied by itching is known as a(n) _____.

9. A(n) _____ is a plugged skin pore.

10. One type of sebaceous cyst is called a _____.

11. Bacterial infection of the nails is called a(n) _____.

12. A common mechanical injury caused by scraping away the skin surface is called a(n) _____.

Using the words in the list, complete the following statements:

avulsion	ephelis
blunt trauma	nevus
laceration	hirsutism
vesicles	alopecia
pressure ulcer	hemangioma
hematoma	"cradle cap"

13. A(n) _____ occurs when a portion of skin or an appendage is pulled or torn away.

14. A cut in the skin caused by a sharp object such as a knife, razor, or glass is known medically as a(n) _____.

15. When an individual is struck by an item such as a hammer or club or is thrown into an object like a steering wheel or wall, the individual may sustain a _____ _____ injury.

16. _____ are fluid-filled circumscribed elevations.

17. A decubitus ulcer is also called a(n) _____.

18. A large bruise is called a(n) _____.

19. A(n) _____ is a freckle.

20. A(n) _____ is the same as a mole.

21. _____ is excessive hair growth.

22. Complete or partial hair loss is called _____.

23. A benign tumor of the blood vessels is called a(n) _____.

24. Infant seborrheic dermatitis is called _____.

Using the words in the list, complete the following statements:

chicken pox	verrucae
epidermis	urticaria
erysipelas	shingles
folliculitis	lice
frostbite	keloid
herpes simplex 2	jock itch

25. Hives are also called _____.

26. Tinea cruris is commonly known as _____.

27. A strep cellulitis of the face or legs is called _____.

28. Pediculosis is also called _____.

29. Inflammation and infection of a hair follicle is _____.

30. Herpes zoster is also known as _____.

31. Herpes varicella is commonly called _____.

32. The _____ is the outer layer of skin.

33. _____ are also known as warts.

34. Genital herpes is also known as _____.

35. A(n) _____ is a raised, firm, irregular-shaped mass of scar tissue that develops following trauma or surgical incision.

36. Freezing of tissue usually on the face, fingers, toes, and ears is called _____.

Short Answer

Provide answers to the following:

1. Describe the skin.

    _____

    _____

    _____

    _____

2. List the common signs and symptoms of skin problems.

    _____

    _____

3. What are the various types of herpes?

    a. _____

    b. _____

    c. _____

    d. _____

True/False

_____ 1. Research conducted on botanicals revealed that none of them have a positive effect on skin conditions.

_____ 2. Herbs from the Lamiaceae family (mint group) are safe and effective for the treatment of herpes simplex virus.

_____ 3. Using sunscreen with an SPF of 30 or higher on all exposed skin is recommended to prevent sunburn.

_____ 4. Using tanning beds is a good method for tanning the skin without harm.

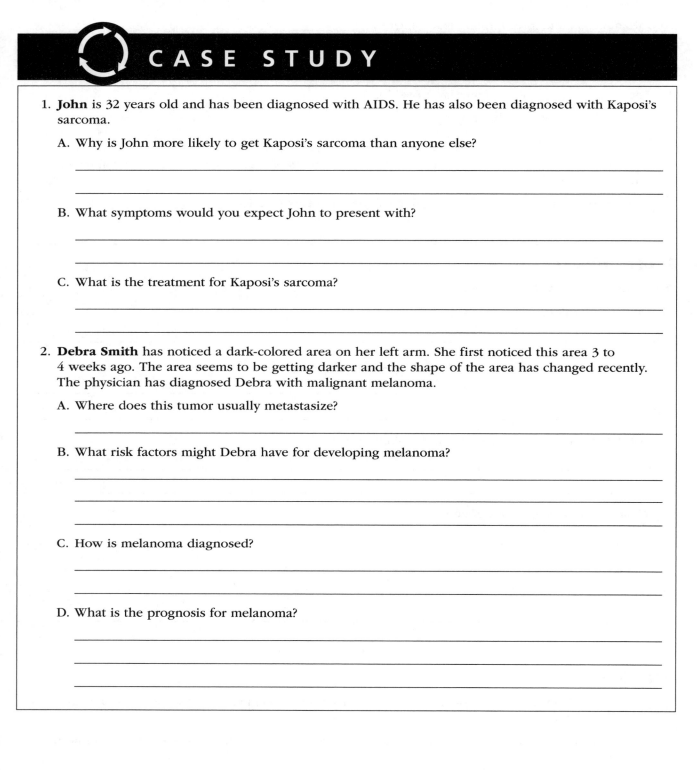

C A S E   S T U D Y

1. **John** is 32 years old and has been diagnosed with AIDS. He has also been diagnosed with Kaposi's sarcoma.

   A. Why is John more likely to get Kaposi's sarcoma than anyone else?

   _____

   _____

   B. What symptoms would you expect John to present with?

   _____

   _____

   C. What is the treatment for Kaposi's sarcoma?

   _____

   _____

2. **Debra Smith** has noticed a dark-colored area on her left arm. She first noticed this area 3 to 4 weeks ago. The area seems to be getting darker and the shape of the area has changed recently. The physician has diagnosed Debra with malignant melanoma.

   A. Where does this tumor usually metastasize?

   _____

   B. What risk factors might Debra have for developing melanoma?

   _____

   _____

   _____

   C. How is melanoma diagnosed?

   _____

   _____

   D. What is the prognosis for melanoma?

   _____

   _____

   _____

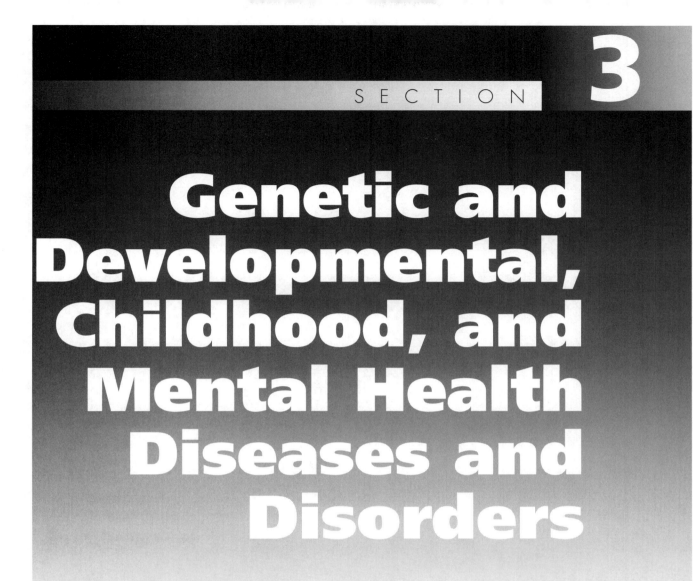

Genetic and Developmental, Childhood, and Mental Health Diseases and Disorders

Genetic and Developmental Diseases and Disorders

Define Terms

Define the following terms:

1. anomaly _____

   _____

2. atresia _____

   _____

3. dystrophy _____

   _____

4. autosome _____

   _____

5. congenital _____

   _____

6. dominant _____

   _____

7. exocrine _____

   _____

8. gene _____

   _____

9. genotype _____

   _____

10. somatic _____

    _____

Matching Terms

Match the following terms with the correct definition:

_____ 1. buccal smear

_____ 2. epicanthus

_____ 3. heterozygous

_____ 4. karyotyping

_____ 5. microcephaly

A. having different paired genes

B. a test for evaluating chromosomes utilizing cells from the mouth

C. a unit on the chromosome

D. a method of identifying chromosomes

E. a fold of skin across the medial aspect of the eye

F. an abnormally small head

Match the following terms with the correct definition:

_____ 6. mitosis

_____ 7. recessive

_____ 8. stricture

_____ 9. viscous

_____ 10. pyloromyotomy

A. reproduction of cells that yields identical daughter cells

B. thick

C. weak, lacks control

D. surgery on a sphincter muscle of the stomach

E. narrowing

F. part of the chromosome carrying DNA

Define Abbreviations

Define the following abbreviations:

1. FAS _____

2. PKU _____

3. CP _____

4. CHD _____

5. MD _____

Identify Diagnostic Tests

Identify the following diagnostic tests:

1. amniotic fluid analysis _____

2. ultrasonography _____

3. muscle biopsy _____

4. electromyography _____

5. blood test for phenylketonuria _____

Condition Table

Complete the following table:

Condition and Definition	Signs and Symptoms	Diagnostic Tests	Treatment Plan
Tay-Sachs Disease			
Fetal Alcohol Syndrome			
Hirschsprung's Disease			
Down Syndrome			
Phenylketonuria			
Failure to Thrive			
Imperforate Anus			
Cleft Palate			
Tetralogy of Fallot			
Meckel's Diverticulum			

Completion

Using the words in the list, complete the following statements:

anomaly

blue babies

congenital

murmur

microcephaly

karyotyping

auscultation

dominant

germ cells

phenotype

imperforate anus

Meckel's diverticulum

1. Babies born with tetralogy of Fallot are called _____ _____.

2. An abnormality is known as a(n) _____.

3. A condition a person is born with is known as _____.

4. An abnormal heart sound is called a(n) _____.

5. _____ is a small brain.

6. The process of visualizing chromosomes is called _____.

7. _____ is listening to the chest with a stethoscope.

8. A gene in control is a _____ gene.

9. _____ are also called sex cells.

10. The expression of a trait such as brown hair or blue eyes is called a(n) _____.

11. Failure of the anus to connect to the rectum is called _____ _____.

12. Outpouching of the diverticulum of the ileum is known as _____ _____.

Using the words in the list, complete the following statements:

coarctation of the aorta	cleft lip
phenylketonuria	chordee
failure to thrive	hydrocephalus
talipes equinovarus	atrial septal defect
Tay–Sachs disease	FAS
anencephaly	atresia
gene	

13. _____ _____ is the narrowing of the descending thoracic aorta.

14. A congenital fissure in the lip is called a(n) _____ _____.

15. Faulty protein metabolism causes a disease called _____.

16. Abnormal downward curvature of the penis is known as _____.

17. _____ _____ _____ is lack of physical growth and development in an infant or a child.

18. _____ is fluid on the brain.

19. Clubfoot is known medically as _____ _____.

20. An opening between the right and left atria is called _____ _____ _____.

21. _____ _____ is an error in lipid metabolism and results in an accumulation of toxins in the brain.

22. The abbreviation for fetal alcohol syndrome is _____.

23. Severe congenital malformation resulting in the absence of the brain or cranial vault is called _____.

24. Congenital absence or closure of a normal opening or lumen in the body is known as _____.

25. A(n) _____ is an ultramicroscopic unit of DNA.

Short Answer

Provide answers to the following:

1. Describe chromosomes.

_____

_____

_____

_____

2. Describe how genetic disorders are passed to offspring from parents.

a. _____

b. _____

c. _____

d. _____

3. What are the causes of congenital anomalies?

a. _____

b. _____

c. _____

d. _____

True/False

_____ 1. A mixture from several plants called Ankaferd Blood Stopper (ABS) has been used in Turkey for hundreds of years as a treatment for bleeding disorders.

_____ 2. ABS has had therapeutic effects on wound healing and has also shown some anti-infective and antineoplastic properties.

_____ 3. A new gene therapy that causes the liver to develop more of clotting factor IX is being tested and shows promising results.

_____ 4. In the hereditary disease, hemophilia B, the blood does not clot properly due to a lack of clotting factor VI.

_____ 5. Patients with hemophilia B must receive the clotting factor by oral tablets given daily.

⟳ CASE STUDY

Mr. and Mrs. Pearson have three children who are grown. Two years ago, they were surprised when they found out Mrs. Pearson was pregnant again. After birth, their daughter Casey was diagnosed with Down syndrome. She is a loving child but does have some limitations.

What are some of the typical signs of Down syndrome?

_____

_____

_____

_____

_____

_____

_____

Childhood Diseases and Disorders

Define Terms

Define the following terms:

1. incubation period _____

   _____

2. malaise _____

   _____

3. Koplik's spots _____

   _____

4. rhinitis _____

   _____

5. catarrhal _____

   _____

6. paroxysmal _____

   _____

7. pyoderma _____

   _____

8. inspiratory stridor _____

   _____

9. supine _____

   _____

10. prone _____

    _____

11. colic _____

    _____

12. intrathecal _____

    _____

13. exudates _____

    _____

14. flatulence _____

_____

15. nits _____

_____

Matching Terms

Match the following terms with the correct definition:

_____ 1. dormant   A. a sense of well-being

_____ 2. encephalopathy   B. surgical removal of the adenoids

_____ 3. euphoric   C. state of being inactive

_____ 4. orchitis   D. inflammation of the testis

_____ 5. adenoidectomy   E. disease of the brain

                                     F. listening to the heart with a stethoscope

Match the following terms with the correct definition:

_____ 6. tonsillectomy   A. blister-like eruptions on the skin

_____ 7. vesicles   B. producing psychedelic alterations in function

_____ 8. patent   C. salivary glands

_____ 9. hallucinogenic   D. surgery to remove tissue in the nasopharynx

_____ 10. parotid glands   E. open

                                     F. a state of ill feeling

Define Abbreviations

Define the following abbreviations:

1. AIDS _____

2. HIV _____

3. SIDS _____

4. TB _____

5. MMR _____

6. DTP–Hib _____

Identify Diagnostic Tests

Identify the following diagnostic tests:

1. chest X-ray _____

2. sputum culture _____

3. skin tests _____

4. throat culture _____

5. stool examination _____

6. pulmonary function tests _____

7. bone scan _____

8. bone marrow biopsy _____

9. complete blood count _____

10. audiometry _____

Condition Table

Complete the following table:

Condition and Definition	Signs and Symptoms	Diagnostic Tests	Treatment Plan
Tonsillitis			
Sudden Infant Death Syndrome			
Measles			
Mumps			
Rubella			
Pertussis			
Diphtheria			
AIDS			
Croup			
Tuberculosis			

Completion

Using the words in the list, complete the following statements:

rubeola	mumps
whooping cough	orchitis
influenza	Koplik's spots
flatulence	catarrhal
vesicles	malaise

1. Another name for measles is _____.

2. Pertussis is also called _____.

3. An infection of the parotid glands is known as _____.

4. An inflammation of the testes is called _____.

5. _____ is more commonly called the flu.

6. _____ are unique to measles and are often the definitive symptom that makes the diagnosis.

7. _____ is excessive gas.

8. _____ are blister-like eruptions on the skin.

9. Inflammation of the nasal mucous membranes is called _____.

10. _____ is a feeling of general discomfort.

Using the words in the list, complete the following statements:

dormant	paroxysmal
incubation period	prone
inspiratory stridor	strabismus
laryngotracheobronchitis	supine
nits	tularemia

11. The _____ _____ is the time between exposure to the disease and the presence of the symptoms.

12. _____ _____ is a high-pitched sound during inspiration due to a blocked airway.

13. A _____ attack is a spasm or convulsion.

14. _____ is the state of being inactive.

15. _____ are lice eggs.

16. _____ is lying face down.

17. _____ is lying face up.

18. Rabbit fever is also known as _____.

19. _____ is also known as croup.

20. A crossed or lazy eye is called _____.

Short Answer

Provide answers to the following:

1. What is the recommended schedule for immunizations for children?

_____

_____

_____

_____

_____

_____

_____

2. Describe some important points about respiratory diseases in children.

_____

_____

_____

_____

_____

3. Describe some important points about fungal diseases in children.

_____

_____

_____

_____

_____

4. Describe some important points about digestive diseases in children.

_____

_____

_____

_____

_____

5. Describe some important points about viral diseases in children.

_____

_____

_____

_____

_____

True/False

_____ 1. Many children are taking immunosuppressive medications after organ transplantation or for other diseases.

_____ 2. New research is finding that immunosuppressive medications might also cause increased responses to the routine immunizations a child receives.

_____ 3. The new recommendation is to administer immunizations a month after taking immunosuppressive medications whenever possible.

_____ 4. Research has shown that the immune system is not vulnerable to the environmental changes that have occurred in recent decades.

_____ 5. Some plants commonly found in the home can be toxic to children.

_____ 6. Child-resistant packaging does not mean childproof packaging.

_____ 7. The meningococcal vaccine is only recommended for adults.

_____ 8. The varicella vaccine is given to prevent chickenpox.

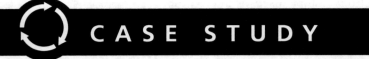

CASE STUDY

Nancy is the mother of Jamie, a toddler who seems to be very curious. Nancy is concerned about the safety of her home with a toddler who is very active and can wander throughout the one-level home rather easily. Besides putting all medicines, cosmetics, and plants out of Jamie's reach, what other tips should Nancy know about preventing poisonings in children?

_____

_____

_____

_____

_____

_____

_____

CHAPTER 21

Mental Health Diseases and Disorders

Define Terms

Define the following terms:

1. addiction _____
   _____

2. affect _____
   _____

3. bulimia _____
   _____

4. delirium tremens _____
   _____

5. circadian rhythms _____
   _____

6. delusions _____
   _____

7. dependency _____
   _____

8. intoxicated _____
   _____

9. mania _____
   _____

10. tolerance _____
    _____

Matching Terms

Match the following terms with the correct definition:

____   1. obsession

____   2. organic

____   3. dementia

____   4. enuresis

____   5. tic

A. progressive deterioration of mental abilities

B. related to an organ or a physical component

C. sudden, rapid muscle movement or vocalization

D. hyperactivity disorder

E. commonly called *bedwetting*

F. repetition of a thought or an emotion

Match the following terms with the correct definition:

____   6. narcotics

____   7. psychosis

____   8. schizophrenia

____   9. grandiose

____ 10. malingering

A. depressants used as analgesics or painkillers

B. disintegration of one's personality and loss of contact with reality

C. fictitious display of symptoms in order to gain a reward

D. "split mind," a serious mental condition

E. inflated sense of self-worth

F. suspicious actions and feelings

Define Abbreviations

Define the following abbreviations:

1. OCD _____

2. PTSD _____

3. SAD _____

4. ADHD _____

5. LSD _____

6. DTs _____

Condition Table

Complete the following table:

Condition and Definition	Signs and Symptoms	Diagnostic Tests	Treatment Plan
Anorexia			
Bulimia			
Autism			
Schizophrenia			

Intellectual Disability			
Attention-Deficit Hyperactivity Disorder			
Alcoholism			
Depression			
Seasonal Affective Disorder			
Personality Disorders			
Munchausen Syndrome			
Bipolar Disease			

Completion

Using the words in the list, complete the following statements:

delusion	addiction
intoxication	affective disorders
mania	organic
tolerance	withdrawal
tics	bedwetting
psychoses	jealousy
narcolepsy	

1. A false belief that is firmly adhered to although it is not shared by others is a _____.

2. _____ is the physical or psychological dependence on a substance.

3. _____ a daily uncontrollable attack of sleep.

4. _____ occurs when blood alcohol levels reach 0.10% or more.

5. Disorders that involve emotions are called _____ _____.

6. Extreme elation or agitation is known as _____.

7. Mental disorders with some type of known physical cause are called _____.

8. _____ is the ability to endure large amounts of a substance without an adverse effect.

9. The occurrence of unpleasant physical and psychological effects resulting from stopping the use of a substance after the individual is addicted is called _____.

10. _____ are sudden, rapid muscle movements or vocalizations.

11. _____ is medically known as enuresis.

12. _____ are characterized by a disintegration of one's personality and loss of contact with reality.

13. _____ (one type) is the belief that one's sexual partner is unfaithful.

Using the words in the list, complete the following statements:

exhibitionism	voyeurism
grief	transvestic
histrionic	schizophrenia
multiple	schizoid
narcolepsy	panic disorder
paranoid	winter
pedophilia	

14. "Split mind" or split personality is also known as _____.

15. Seasonal affective disorder is also known as _____ depression.

16. A _____ _____ is also called a panic attack.

17. Individuals exhibiting two or more distinct personalities are said to have _____ personalities.

18. A _____ personality exhibits traits of jealousy, suspicion, envy, and hypersensitivity.

19. Loners have _____ personalities.

20. Individuals with a _____ personality may be overly dramatic with expressions of their emotions.

21. _____ occurs when males expose their genitals to an unsuspecting female.

22. The person who is aroused by cross-dressing is said to have _____ fetishism.

23. The disorder when a person is sexually aroused by children is called _____.

24. _____ involves arousal by secretly watching others undress or engage in sexual activity; individuals with this condition are often called "peeping Toms."

25. Daily uncontrollable attack of sleep is called _____.

26. _____ is the natural process of coping with loss.

Short Answer

Provide answers to the following:

1. What are some common signs and symptoms of mental health disorders?

_____

_____

_____

2. What are some categories of common mental health disorders?

_____

_____

_____

3. What are some genetic and acquired causes of intellectual disability?

Genetic: _____

_____

Acquired: _____

_____

True/False

_____ 1. Alcohol affects the teenage brain differently than the adult brain.

_____ 2. The Centers for Disease Control and Prevention (CDC) has reported that 25% of teens use alcohol and participate in binge drinking.

_____ 3. Family therapy may be an effective alternative treatment for drug abuse in adolescents and adults.

_____ 4. Abuse of opium-based drugs is decreasing because researchers have found effective treatment measures.

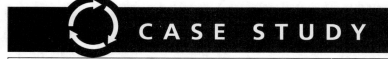

CASE STUDY

Jeffrey is a 43-year-old male who was recently laid off from his job in the auto industry. His wife is concerned that he will become clinically depressed if he cannot get back to work soon.

What are some of the characteristics of depression that Jeffrey's wife might observe?

_____

_____

_____

_____